Yoga for Children

Yoga for Children

Stella Weller

Thorsons
An Imprint of HarperCollins*Publishers*

Thorsons
An Imprint of HarperCollins*Publishers*
77–85 Fulham Palace Road,
Hammersmith, London W6 8JB
1160 Battery Street,
San Francisco,California 94111–1213

Published by Thorsons 1996

1 3 5 7 9 10 8 6 4 2

© Stella Weller asserts the moral right to
be identified as the author of this work

A catalogue record for this book is
available from the British Library

ISBN 0 7225 3206 7

Printed in Great Britain by
Scotprint Ltd, Musselburgh

To David and Karl

Contents

Acknowledgements

Many thanks to everyone who helped me with this book. I am particularly grateful to my husband, Walter, to Erica Smith, to Wanda Whiteley, Linda Mellor and the editorial staff and the design team at Thorsons, and to Jane Bowden for her splendid drawings.

List of Illustrations

Breathing Exercises

Introduction:

To Parents and Teachers

WHEN YOU INTRODUCE YOGA to the children in your care, as part of a fitness programme, you are giving them the chance to learn a discipline which could help to lay a solid foundation for life.

Educators believe that children must be of sound body in order to be sound of mind. They find that children can learn, through practising individually as well as in groups, certain exercises and activities which will help them to acquire invaluable attributes. These include self-awareness (as opposed to self-consciousness in the generally accepted sense), self-discipline, poise, self-reliance and respect for themselves and others.

Regular practice of yoga fosters, early in life, an awareness of what is happening inside as well as outside oneself. This can lead to the following benefits:

- It encourages attentiveness, thus developing and improving concentration.
- It promotes clear thinking and so facilitates learning.
- It fuels the imagination, thereby enhancing creativity.
- It builds self-confidence and therefore contributes to developing and maintaining a positive self-image.
- It promotes harmony between mind and body, and so helps in making appropriate responses to emotional stimuli.
- It reduces health problems.

These benefits accrue, over time, through the practice of techniques that include slow stretching, strengthening movements which are characteristic of yoga postures (exercises or *asanas*), synchronized with breathing, and with full attention given to what is being done. Many of the postures offer an opportunity for the physical expression of mental imagery, with which children are usually very comfortable. They also provide a means whereby those who are shy, withdrawn, or in some way handicapped, can shed their inhibitions and experience a sense of liberty. This satisfies the need for expression: children do not, as a rule, possess the verbal resources which adults generally have. When they are given a chance to release their emotions through physical outlets, they grow creatively. Yoga provides such channels, which are superb for cultivating a strong sense of self-assurance and self-worth.

Children usually tend to have a short attention span and sometimes frequent changes of mood, coupled with a high level of activity. The balancing postures and breathing exercises are especially effective in promoting keen concentration and calm, and in improving co-ordination. The breathing exercises, moreover, are an excellent tool for coping with disorders such as asthma and anxiety states.

The relaxation techniques, both local and general, help in effective stress management: in the maintenance of composure when under pressure. They are also useful for combating insomnia and ensuring sound, refreshing sleep.

Visualization practices offer a safe, enjoyable opportunity for youngsters to give free rein to their imagination. They also maximize the mind's potential for envisioning relaxing images. Researchers have found that visualization complemented other relaxation techniques to facilitate learning, improve concentration, motivation and self-confidence, thereby fostering a positive self-image and reducing health problems.

Yoga postures are done slowly and with awareness, held still for a period of time, and then released. Multiple, random repetitions are not yoga. Variations of the basic exercises can be practised, however, to present challenge, give a sense of individuality, and enhance feelings of achievement, self-confidence and self-worth. They are an excellent complement to the strengths developed through competitive sports. From the most competition-oriented person to the least athletically inclined, yoga has something for everyone.

Many children in the Western world are now spending hour upon hour sitting before television sets and computer screens. They are being driven to and from school and after-school activities, and they are walking far less than children did many years ago. Consequently, even if they engage in outdoor physical activities, they risk early loss of flexibility and may therefore become more susceptible to injuries, aches and pains. Regular yoga practice can help to prevent this, and also enable them to become fitter and less tense and anxious. The slow-moving, leisurely stretching and strengthening exercises can be done even where space is limited. They are ideal for maintaining firm muscles and flexible joints, and for promoting good postural habits.

Encouraging the incorporation of yoga techniques into daily routines is one of the best things you can do to foster self-discipline and self-responsibility in the children you look after, guide and instruct. Teaching them, early in life, to utilize their own natural, inner resources (physical and mental faculties and breath) to deal with day-to-day situations and with some of life's stressors, in order to be less dependent on external props and aids, is one of the most precious gifts you can offer them.

The practice of yoga is becoming more widespread as people are finally realizing that it is not a religion, and therefore poses no threat to their religious or philosophical beliefs. Despite its roots in the Hindu culture of India, yoga is, in fact, non-sectarian and may be practised with full confidence by anyone. Increasingly, therefore, it is being incorporated into many health-promotion programmes, particularly because of its potential for reducing stress and for helping people to care for themselves in every aspect of their lives.

Yoga for Children is comprehensive and easy to understand. It has been written for children to practise alone, with parents or in a group, and for teenagers as well. But it is also a useful resource for parents, teachers and other educators, for fitness instructors and for health professionals. It is, in fact, for anyone who is interested in the physical and mental well-being of all children.

Chapter one

How Yoga Began

IN INDIA, THOUSANDS OF YEARS AGO, men called *yogis* would sometimes go into the jungle in order to meditate. During the time that they were meditating, they would carefully observe the birds and beasts that lived there. They would study the manner in which these creatures prepared for sleep, and the way in which they awakened: slowly stretching their limbs and bodies without straining. They watched how they continually tuned up their muscles to help to keep themselves alert, agile and strong.

The yogis began to copy some of the postures and movements they saw, and soon they were able to create hundreds of exercises of their own. They called them *asanas*, a word that means 'postures comfortably held'. They gave many of the exercises animal names, such as the cobra, eagle, lion, rabbit and tortoise.

When they practise these exercises regularly, the yogis found that they had plenty of energy and strength for their work, and that they were able to think clearly, concentrate well and keep fit. They shared their knowledge with others, who in turn passed it on to us by means of writing.

Today, these exercises are practised by millions of people – children and adults – all over the world. They are popular because they do not cause injury when they are properly done, they help you to feel relaxed, and they are fun to do.

The ancient yogis were wise, and therefore designed these exercises to be done in a special way, so as to bring excellent health benefits. You do them slowly and attentively. You never strain. You breathe smoothly while doing them, so as to bring a good supply of oxygen to the working muscles. Once a posture is complete, you hold it steady for a short while before going on to the next posture.

Special breathing exercises help to keep your lungs – your whole body, in fact – healthy. They train you to remain calm when you are tense, anxious, or frightened.

You will probally find the visualization part of yoga particularly enjoyable.
Visualization means creating mental pictures. You will find suggestions in the
instructions for each of the postures in this book. Mental images can be very
powerful, as you will find out as you make progress in your yoga practice.
You can use this 'mind power' to help you to build confidence in yourself,
to do well in school and in after-school activities, and to stay healthy.

Now that you have an idea of how yoga began and what it can do for you,
it is time to go on to the next chapter which tells you how to prepare for the
exercises themselves.

Chapter two

Before You Begin

YOGA EXERCISES HAVE BEEN PRACTISED in many countries for a very long time. They are safe when properly done, and they bring excellent results when practised regularly.

The postures in this book have been carefully chosen because they are safe, suitable and enjoyable for children to do. Children as young as six years (and possibly even younger) may practise them with a parent, grandparent, teacher or other adult. I suggest that all children be supervised when first trying the exercises until they understand clearly what to do. Working in a group is the best way to learn yoga principles.

It is always important to follow the instructions carefully. If you have any worries or doubts, please consult a doctor.

When to practise

Older children and teenagers will benefit from doing the exercises daily, if only for ten minutes. Once a week is fine for younger children practising with a grown-up. A session should last as long as everyone is enjoying it, but forty-five minutes (including the relaxation period at the end) should be enough.

Try to do the exercises at about the same time every day or evening. Doing them in the morning helps to make you alert and energetic for your day's work. Practising them in the evening helps you to relax and sleep soundly. Choose the time that is best for *you*. But it is advisable not to do yoga exercises near a mealtime (see *Food and drink*, below).

If you are ill, or have to stop exercising for some other reason, start again in a gradual way, rather than trying to make up for lost time.

Making the time

Many of the exercises can also be done at odd moments during the day. The *Clock* (Figures 3 to 6) and *Palming* (Figure 61), for example, can be practised in between classes at school, to give your eyes a rest and to relax them. *Figure-Eight* (Figure 1), *Shoulder Rotation* (Figure 2), *Chest Expander* (Figure 33) and *Cow Head* (Figure 36) are excellent for relieving tension in your neck, shoulders and upper back, after bending over a desk or sitting in front of a computer for a long time.

Whenever you feel anxious, practise the *Calming Breath*, which is the first exercise described in the section called 'Breathing Exercises'. You can also practise the *Complete Breath* (Figures 77 and 78) whenever you feel tense.

Food and drink

It is best to do yoga postures on an empty stomach, such as before breakfast or supper. You may practise about two hours after eating a meal or one hour after a light snack. Try not to eat for half an hour after exercising.

Where to practise

The marvellous thing about yoga is that you can practise it in a number of places indoors or outdoors, and even where space is limited. Also, you do not need any special equipment: your breath, your body and your attention are all you need.

There should be enough fresh air in the place you choose to practise. Dim lights are better than bright ones, but you should be able to see clearly.

The floor or ground should be level and smooth. If it is not carpeted, put down a mat or other covering that does not skid, on which to exercise. You can also practise on a grassy surface. The area on which you practise will be called the 'mat' in the exercise instructions.

Comfort and safety

Always make yourself comfortable before starting yoga practice. Go to the toilet and empty your bladder; also your bowel if possible. You may take a warm (*not* hot) shower or bath. Rinsing your mouth or brushing your teeth is also a good idea. (You could also have a bath or shower about fifteen minutes after exercising.)

Wear loose, comfortable clothing which allows you to stretch and breathe easily. Remove hairgrips, jewellery, glasses and any other object that could hurt you while you are exercising. Practise with bare feet whenever you can. Have a light blanket handy, or a cardigan and warm socks ready to put on when you are resting at the end of your exercise session. It is important to remember that girls should *not* practise the *Candle* (Figure 31), the *Half-Candle* (Figure 50) and the *Wheelbarrow* (Figure 76) when they are having a period (i.e. no inverted postures).

How to practise

Yoga exercises are done slowly and smoothly. You breathe regularly while doing them, and you pay strict attention to each movement. In general, you do each posture once only. You then stay in the posture for several seconds to start with, while breathing smoothly. Very young children working with a parent should hold a position for a very short time (about two breaths in and out). As you advance in your practice, you can stay in the posture longer. When you are ready to return to your starting position, you do so slowly and smoothly. Afterwards, you rest for a short while before going on to the next exercise.

Best order

Usually, a forward-bending posture such as the *Curl-Up* (Figure 40) is followed by a posture that stretches the body in the opposite direction, such as the *Bridge* (Figure 29). In the sideward-bending exercises such as the *Triangle* (Figure 72), you repeat the bend to the other side. You do the same with the *Twist* (Figures 73 and 74); you twist to the other side. In the balancing postures such as the *Tree* (Figures 70 and 71), you stand first on one foot and then on the other.

Warming up

Dancers always stretch their arms, legs and body before they begin to dance. This warms them up and makes them limber so that they can dance with grace and excellence. Pianists play scales and exercises to remove stiffness from their wrists, hands and fingers, and to help them to concentrate and not make mistakes. Athletes and sports players also 'warm up' before starting. In the same way, it is very important for you to prepare your body and your mind for doing the yoga exercises. Warm-ups help to prevent muscle pulls and strains as you do the postures themselves, and they enable you to give them the attention they require.

Images

Imagery or visualization is a very important part of yoga practice. It means the forming of mental pictures; seeing with your 'mind's eye', so to speak. When you do each exercise, make a mental picture of the completed posture, and set this as your goal. Be patient with yourself; try not to rush. When you stretch your back, for example, try to imagine it becoming stronger and more supple. When you do breathing exercises, try to imagine bad things, such as sadness and anger, going out of your body as you breathe out. As you breathe in, try to imagine good things, such as happiness and love, coming into your body. Use mental pictures with which you are comfortable and therefore enjoy. Visualization adds enjoyment to yoga practice and improves your concentration.

Creating mental pictures also allows younger children working with a parent or teacher a chance to give free rein to their imagination and let off steam while having a great deal of fun. They can, for example, hiss like a snake when doing the *Cobra* (Figure 34), caw like a *Crow* (Figure 38) or roar like a *Lion* (Figure 55).

Breathing

Breathe smoothly in and out of your nostrils, unless the exercise instructions tell you differently. Match your breathing to the movement you are doing; it should feel natural. *Do not* hold your breath. Breathing as you exercise brings oxygen to feed your working muscles and takes away wastes from your body.

Cooling down

End each exercise period, no matter how short it is, with relaxation. Most yoga classes finish with *Complete Relaxation* (Figure 35), but you may prefer just to sit quietly for a few minutes in one of the *Lotus* postures (Figures 56 to 58) or in the *Japanese Sitting Position* (Figures 51 and 52) with your eyes closed, concentrating on your breathing until it is slow and smooth. Cover yourself with a light blanket, or put on something warm if you begin to feel cold. (See the section on *Comfort and safety*, page 4). When you feel rested, you can then end your exercise period.

Chapter three

Warm-ups

SOME OF THE WARM-UP EXERCISES in this section can be done during the day, at school or wherever you do most of your work. They can even be done during the commercial breaks while you watch television! You will find them useful not only for warming up your body before the main exercises (postures), but also for preventing tension from building up, so that you do not become too anxious or afraid about things.

Parents and grandparents can make a game of practising warm-ups with small children to stop them from becoming bored and irritable. Teachers can stop a class when children's attention strays and spend a few moments practising appropriate exercises together.

FIGURE-EIGHT

How to do it
1. Sit tall. Keep your hands and shoulders still. Close your eyes or keep them open. Breathe slowly and smoothly.
2. Imagine a large figure-eight lying on its side in front of you. With your nose, mouth or face, pretend to draw the figure-eight in the air, starting with a clockwise motion (Figure 1). Do so *slowly and smoothly* at least five times.
3. Repeat step 2, starting with an anti-clockwise motion, the same number of times. Remember to keep breathing slowly and smoothly.
4. Rest.

What it does
The *Figure-Eight* exercise is superb for preventing your neck from becoming tense, and may even help to prevent a headache.

Special notes
Do the *Figure-Eight* exercise in between classes at school, during your lunch break, or while waiting for your transport home. If you do not wish anyone to see you doing it, practise it in the cloakroom at school, for example, or in the privacy of your own room at home.

You may also do this exercise while standing.

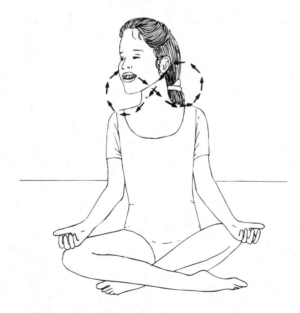

Figure 1 Figure-eight

SHOULDER ROTATION

How to do it.
1. Sit tall. Keep your hands still. Close your eyes or keep them open. Breathe slowly and smoothly.
2. Pretend to draw circles with your shoulders (Figure 2). Do this at least five times in a forwards-to-backwards direction. Do so slowly and smoothly.
3. Make imaginary circles with your shoulders in the opposite direction, that is, backwards-to-forwards, at least five times. Remember to keep breathing slowly and smoothly.
4. Rest.

What it does
Rotating your shoulders helps to remove tension from your shoulders and upper back. Do it after or before the *Figure-Eight* neck warm-up, as the two exercises reinforce each other.

Special notes
Practise rotating your shoulders in spare moments in between classes at school, and while doing chores at home. If you do not wish anyone to see you doing it, find a private place to practise in.

You may do this warm-up while standing as well as sitting. Try to practise it while taking a warm shower; it feels so good!

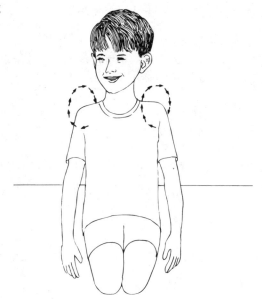

Figure 2 Shoulder Rotation

CLOCK

How to do it

1. Sit tall. Keep your head, shoulders and hands still. Breathe slowly and smoothly.
2. Imagine looking at a large clock in front of you. Look at number twelve (Figure 3) for one second (mentally count 'one thousand', that is one second). Now look at number one on the clock face then two. Look at three (Figure 4); look at each number for one second. Continue in this way until you reach six (Figure 5). Go on to seven and eight; then nine (Figure 6). Proceed to ten and eleven. Finish with twelve (Figure 3). Remember to keep breathing slowly and smoothly.
3. Look straight ahead.
4. Repeat step 2, going in the opposite direction (anti-clockwise) this time.
5. Look straight ahead. Gently blink several times. Close your eyes and rest them. Keep breathing slowly and smoothly.

What it does

The *Clock* helps to strengthen your eye muscles and to keep your eyes healthy. It relieves eye strain, which may sometimes occur after doing a great deal of eye work, such as reading fine print, especially in poor light. Eye strain can also be a result of spending a great deal of time in front of a computer screen.

Blinking gently bathes your eyes with their natural fluid and brightens them. It helps you to see more clearly.

Special notes

Take breaks from reading, watching television or sitting in front of a computer screen to practise the *Clock*.

Practise these exercises outdoors whenever you can, to benefit from the fresh air as well.

Palming (Figure 61) is a good exercise to do following the *Clock*.

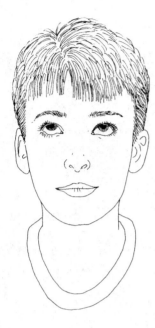

Figure 3 Clock (1)

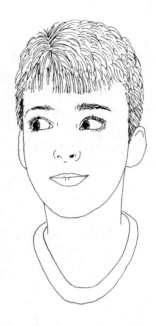

Figure 4 Clock (2)

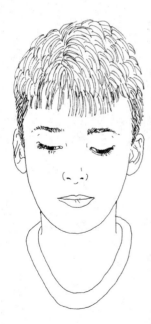

Figure 5 Clock (3)

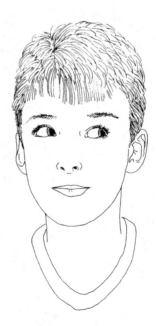

Figure 6 Clock (4)

BUTTERFLY

How to do it
1. Sit tall. Breathe slowly and smoothly.
2. Bend one leg and then the other, bringing the soles of your feet together. Bring your feet close to your body.
3. Clasp your hands around your feet.
4. Pretend that your folded legs are a butterfly's wings. Flap them down and up, again and again (Figure 7).
5. Stretch out your legs and rest.

What it does
The *Butterfly* keeps your hip, knee and ankle joints flexible. It also stretches the muscles of your inner thighs and keeps them firm and healthy. These muscles bring your thighs together. When they are shortened, the hips are rigid and any activity requiring you to spread out the legs, such as horse riding, becomes difficult.

The *Butterfly* is a very good warm-up to do before practising the *Lotus* postures (Figures 56 to 58), the *Archer* (Figure 27), the *Star* (Figure 66) and the *Tortoise* (Figure 69).

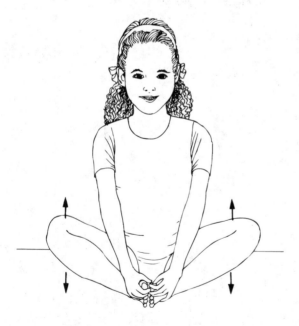

Figure 7 Butterfly

ANKLE ROTATION

How to do it
1. Sit tall, on a chair, bench or stool – anywhere that allows you to move your feet freely. Breathe slowly and smoothly.
2. Make imaginary circles with your feet, clockwise, as many times as you wish (Figure 8). Do so slowly.
3. Rotate your ankles in the opposite direction, that is, anti-clockwise. (If you prefer, you may rotate your right ankle clockwise while rotating your left ankle anti-clockwise, i.e. both ankles rotating outwards, then repeat the circles in the opposite direction, i.e. both rotating inwards.)
4. Rest.

What it does
Rotating your ankles prevents them from becoming stiff, and keeps them, and the feet also, strong and healthy. It is a good exercise to do when your feet are cold; it helps to warm them up.

Special notes
Ankle rotations are good preparation for all the standing exercises, such as the *Eagle* (Figures 44 and 45), and for the *Squat* (Figure 65). They are also good to do when you prepare for outdoor activities, such as cycling and walking (and also skiing).

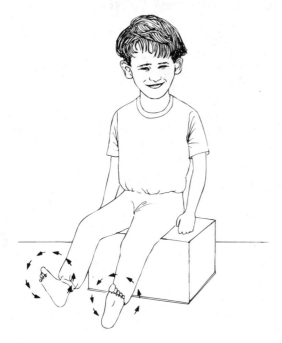

Figure 8 Ankle Rotation

ROCKING HORSE

How to do it

1. Sit on a carpeted floor, exercise mat or grassy surface. (From now on, I shall call this surface the 'mat'.) Bend your legs and rest the soles of your feet flat on the mat. Bring your legs close to your body.
2. Pass your arms under your knees and hug your thighs. Tilt your head down and tuck in your chin. Make your back as round as you can. Breathe slowly and smoothly.
3. Breathe in (inhale) and kick backwards to help you to roll onto your back (Figure 9).
4. Breathe out (exhale) and kick forwards to come up again into a sitting position. *Be careful* not to land heavily onto your feet as this may hurt your spine. Try instead to touch the mat lightly with your feet or toes.
5. Repeat steps 3 and 4 again and again, like a rocking horse rocking to and fro; back and forth. Keep breathing smoothly.
6. Rest.

What it does

The *Rocking Horse* is wonderful for massaging your back and for warming up your whole body. It is excellent for keeping your abdominal (tummy) muscles firm and healthy. It prevents your hamstring muscles (at the back of your legs) from becoming short and tight. It is good for improving your co-ordination.

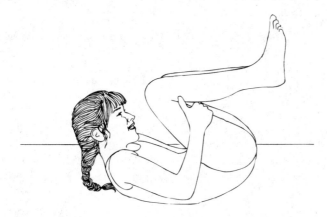

Figure 9 Rocking Horse

Special notes

The *Rocking Horse* is a good warm-up to practise before doing the *Candle* (Figure 31), the *Curl-Up* (Figure 40), the *Half-Candle* (Figure 50) and the *Wheelbarrow* (Figure 76).

Parents can have a lot of fun practising the Rocking Horse with small children, encouraging them to put mental pictures into words, by saying things like, 'Giddy-up, horsie!'.

CAT STRETCH

How to do it

1. Get on your hands and knees and pretend to be a cat (Figure 10). Breathe slowly and smoothly.
2. Exhale (breathe out) and arch your back: make your shoulders round and tuck your bottom down, gently stretching your spine (Figure 11).
3. Inhale (breathe in) and very slowly stretch the front of your body: lift your head high and feel the front of your neck stretch gently. Stretch one leg backwards as far as you can without straining (Figure 12).
4. Exhale and lower your head. Bend the knee of your outstretched leg and bring it in towards your forehead. Feel your back muscles stretching (Figure 13).
5. Inhale and come back to your starting position (Figure 10).
6. Repeat steps 2 to 5; this time stretch out the other leg when you come to step 3 (Figure 12). The two sets of exercises make one 'round'.
7. Repeat the entire exercise, that is, one more round, at least once.
8. Sit or lie down and rest.

What it does

The *Cat Stretch* exercises keep your spine strong and flexible. They help to prevent backache. They improve circulation to every part of your body.

Special notes

Practise the *Cat Stretch* when you get out of bed in the morning to help you to wake up. Practise it at the end of the day to relax your whole body, and to help you to sleep well.

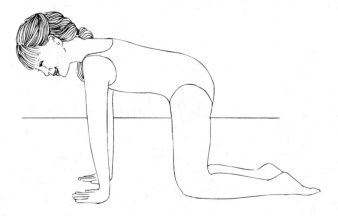

Figure 10 Cat Stretch: starting position

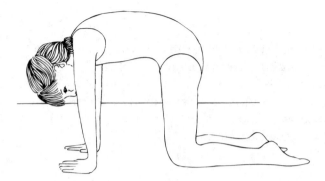

Figure 11 Cat Stretch: arching the back

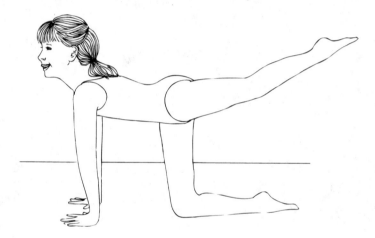

Figure 12 Cat Stretch: leg stretch

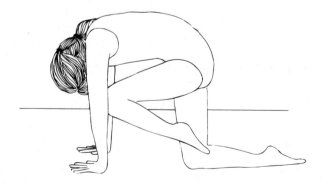

Figure 13 Cat Stretch: knee to forehead

SUN GREETING

How to do it

1. Stand tall, with your body weight equally distributed between your feet. Bring the palms of your hands together in front of your chest (Figure 14). Breathe slowly and smoothly.
2. Inhale, raise your arms, and *carefully* bend backwards to stretch the front of your body; tighten your buttocks as you do so (Figure 15). Imagine welcoming the sun, along with its warmth, energy and brightness.

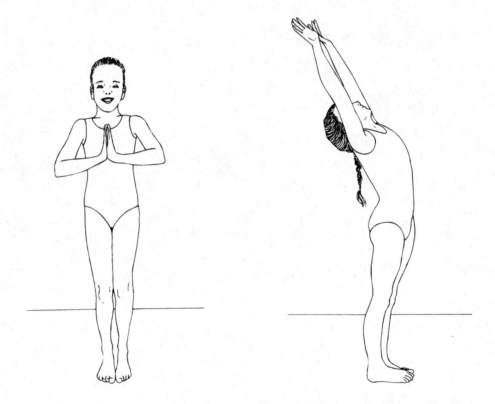

Figure 14 Sun Greeting: starting position　　**Figure 15** Sun Greeting: backward bend

3. Exhale and bend forwards; place your hands on the mat beside your feet (Figure 16). Keep your knees straight if you can. Feel your back stretch; feel the kinks disappearing after a night curled up in bed.
4. Inhale and look up. Keep your hands on the mat and step backwards with your *left* foot; point your toes forwards (Figure 17). Enjoy the delight of your leg muscles stretching.
5. Without either inhaling or exhaling, step backwards with your right foot. Your body should be level from head to heels, like a slide in a playground (Figure 18). Feel energy entering your body.

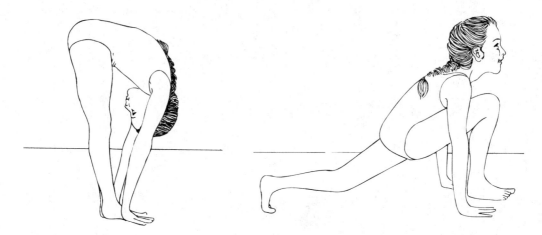

Figure 16 Sun Greeting: forward bend   **Figure 17** Sun Greeting: leg stretch

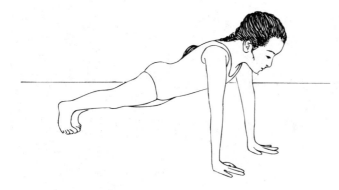

Figure 18 Sun Greeting: slide

6. Exhale as you lower your knees to the mat. Also lower your chin or forehead (whichever is more comfortable) and your chest to the mat. Relax your feet; point your toes backwards (Figure 19).
7. Inhale. Lower your body to the mat and *slowly and carefully* arch your back, waking it up as you uncoil it, like a serpent. Keep your head back and your hands pressed to the mat (Figure 20). This is the *Cobra*, also shown in Figure 34.

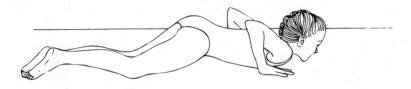

Figure 19 Sun Greeting: knee-chest position

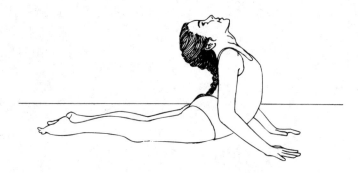

Figure 20 Sun Greeting: cobra

8. Exhale. Point your toes forwards. Push against the mat with your hands to help to raise your hips. Keep your arms straight or almost straight. Hang your head down. Aim your heels towards the mat, but *do not force* them down (Figure 21). This is the *Dog Stretch*, also shown in Figure 43. Feel the wonderful stretch in your arms and legs. Feel your muscles waking up.

9. Inhale, look up, rock forwards onto your toes and step between your hands with your *left* foot (Figure 22).

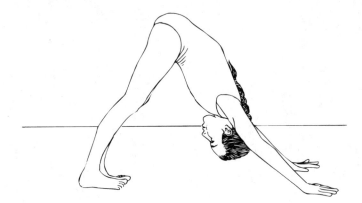

Figure 21 Sun Greeting: dog stretch

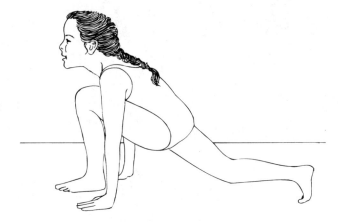

Figure 22 Sun Greeting: forward step

10. Exhale, step between your hands with your other foot and come into a forward-bending position, as you did in step 3 (Figure 23).
11. Inhale, come up carefully into a standing position and move smoothly into a backward-bending position, with arms raised, as you did in step 2 (Figure 24).
12. Exhale and return to your starting position (Figure 25).
13. Relax your arms. Lie down and rest, or do the entire exercise (steps 1 to 12) one or more times. Rest afterwards.

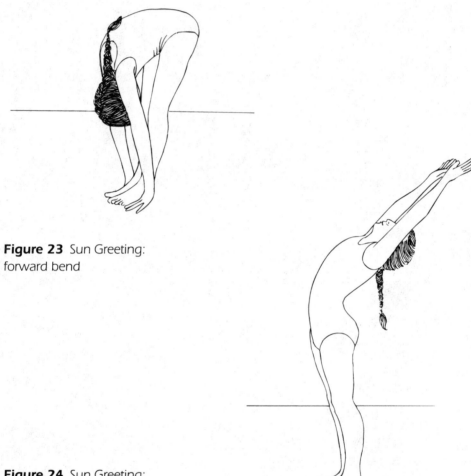

Figure 23 Sun Greeting: forward bend

Figure 24 Sun Greeting: backward bend

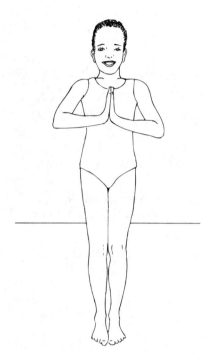

Figure 25 Sun Greeting:
starting position

What it does

The *Sun Greeting* exercises are excellent for helping to keep your body trim, flexible and healthy. They are useful for improving your concentration because you have to pay attention to both your breathing and the movements.

Practised in the morning, these exercises are splendid for waking you up and keeping you alert and energetic. Done at night, they help to relax you so that you can sleep soundly.

On days when you do not have much time, you can practise the *Sun Greeting* exercises as an almost complete exercise session. Add the *Triangle* (Figure 72) and the *Twist* (Figure 73 or 74). Include the *Candle* (Figure 31) or the *Half-Candle* (Figure 50) if you wish.

You may also do each step of the *Sun Greeting* as a separate posture: stay in each position for a few seconds while breathing slowly and smoothly, then move on to the next and do the same. Rest when you have completed all the steps.

The images given in the instructions are only suggestions. You may prefer to use your own. If you think of what the sun brings (warmth, light, energy, good feelings, and so on), it will help you to create your own mental pictures.

𝍅𝍅 𝍅𝍅 𝍅𝍅 𝍅𝍅 𝍅𝍅 𝍅𝍅 𝍅𝍅 𝍅𝍅 𝍅𝍅 𝍅𝍅 𝍅𝍅 𝍅𝍅 𝍅𝍅 𝍅𝍅 𝍅𝍅 𝍅𝍅 𝍅𝍅 𝍅𝍅 𝍅𝍅 𝍅𝍅

Cooling down

Cool-down exercises allow your body to adjust slowly from practising the postures to returning to your usual activities. Except for the *Rocking Horse* (Figure 9), all the exercises in this section may also be used as cool-down exercises. Do them very slowly, and lie down and rest afterwards.

The *Rag Doll* (Figure 63) is another useful cool-down exercise. *Complete Relaxation* (Figure 35) is an excellent way to end your exercise period.

Remember to put on warm socks and a cardigan, or to cover yourself up with a light blanket, when resting at the end of cooling-down exercises. This will stop you from getting cold after you have already cooled down.

Chapter four

Postures

YOGA EXERCISES ARE CALLED POSTURES, POSES OR *ASANAS*. They are safe and enjoyable. The postures are done slowly and gracefully while breathing smoothly. Each completed posture is maintained or 'held' steady for several seconds to start with; longer as you become more comfortable with it. Remember that small children working with parents or teachers should hold a position only for a very short time (about two breaths in and out).

When doing the postures, you need to give them your full attention; otherwise you will not gain all the possible benefits. These are not just physical exercises; they are mental exercises also. They help to develop your ability to concentrate well, and they train you to stay calm when you are under pressure.

Younger children tend to have a short attention span and so learning something new has to be made enjoyable and interesting for them. The postures in this section have therefore been given names which most children will know and understand. Adults working with small children can help them to learn by doing the postures with them, and even making up games from them. Use your imagination and have fun.

ANGLE BALANCE (V-SIT)

How to do it
1. Sit with your legs bent and the soles of your feet flat on the mat. Breathe slowly and smoothly.
2. Tilt backwards so that your feet lift off the mat, and you are balancing on your bottom.
3. Stretch your arms out in front; keep them parallel to the mat.
4. Carefully straighten your legs but *do not strain* (Figure 26). Pay attention to every move you make, to help you to keep your balance.
5. Think of your legs as being one side of a large letter 'V' and your body being the other side. Stay in this posture for as long as you comfortably can. Keep breathing slowly and smoothly.
6. Carefully return to your starting position.
7. Sit or lie down and rest.

What it does
The *Angle Balance* is a very good exercise to do to keep your abdominal (tummy) muscles firm. When these muscles are strong, they give support to your spine and help to prevent back problems.

Because it is a balancing exercise, the *Angle Balance* trains you to concentrate, improves your co-ordination, and helps you to stay calm.

Special note
This exercise is called the *Angle Balance* because your legs and body form an angle, as the letter 'V' does.

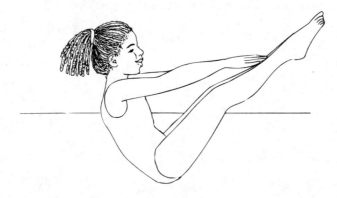

Figure 26 Angle Balance (V-Sit)

ARCHER (SHOOTING BOW)

How to do it
1. Sit tall, with your legs straight out in front of you.
2. Reach out and hold on to both big toes. Breathe slowly and smoothly.
3. Keeping your *left* leg firmly on the mat, and still holding the big toe, bend your *right* leg and *carefully* bring your foot towards your right ear (Figure 27).
4. Pretend to be an archer. Imagine that your left leg is a bow, which you are holding steady. Pretend that your right hand is pulling back the bowstring and arrow. Fix your gaze on an imaginary target in front of you. Stay in this posture for as long as you comfortably can, breathing smoothly.
5. Slowly return to your starting position. Rest for a few seconds.
6. Repeat the exercise, changing hands: hold the 'bow' with your right hand (keeping your right leg on the mat); bend your left leg to pull back on the 'arrow' and 'bowstring' with your left hand.
7. Stay in this posture for as long as you comfortably can.
8. Carefully return to your starting position. Rest.

What it does
The *Archer* exercises all the joints of your arms and legs, and keeps them flexible. It also keeps the arm and leg muscles firm and healthy. This exercise is also good for improving, balance, concentration and co-ordination.

Special notes
Breathing slowly and smoothly, and paying attention to your breathing, will help you to keep your balance while practising the *Archer* and other balancing exercises.

A more challenging version for advanced students is to pull your right foot towards your left ear with your left hand, while holding onto your left big toe with your right hand (the left leg remaining outstretched on the mat). Repeat the exercises, changing hands and feet.

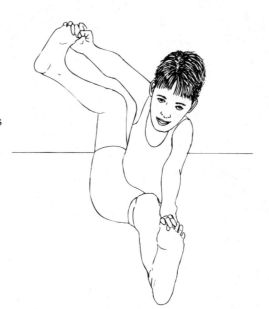

Figure 27 Archer (Shooting Bow)

BOW

How to do it
1. Lie on your front or abdomen (tummy), with your legs slightly apart and your arms at your sides. Breathe slowly and smoothly.
2. Bend your knees and bring your feet close to your bottom.
3. *Carefully* tilt your head back. Reach for your feet; grasp your ankles.
4. Exhale as you push your feet away and up. This action will raise your legs and arch your body (Figure 28).
5. Keep breathing smoothly as you stay in this posture for as long as you comfortably can. Close your eyes if you wish, and pretend to be an archer's bow.
6. Ease yourself back onto the mat, into your starting position. Rest.

What it does
The *Bow* keeps your back muscles strong and your spine flexible. It expands your chest and helps you to breathe more deeply. Deep breathing is good for your health.

Special notes
From the face-down position, push yourself up onto your hands and knees, and rest in the *Curling Leaf* posture (Figure 39) after practising the *Bow*. This will relax your back muscles.

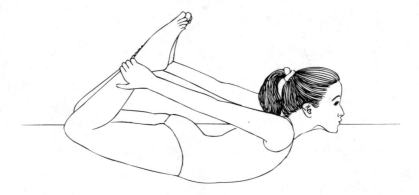

Figure 28 Bow

BRIDGE

How to do it

1. Lie on your back. Bend your legs and rest the soles of your feet flat on the mat, comfortably near your bottom. Place your arms at your sides; turn your palms downwards. Breathe slowly and smoothly.
2. Inhale and raise first your hips, then the rest of your back, in one smooth movement. Keep your arms pressed to the mat. You are now a strong bridge (Figure 29).
3. Stay in this posture for as long as you comfortably can. Keep breathing smoothly.
4. Lower your back to the mat: imagine uncoiling your spine, one bone at a time, onto the mat, starting at the top and working towards the bottom.
5. Stretch out your legs and rest.

What it does

The *Bridge* is a wonderful exercise for toning up the muscles of your back and abdomen (tummy). It keeps your spine flexible and healthy. It gives a good stretch to your whole body.

Special notes

Make yourself into a longer *Bridge* by stretching your arms back over your head. Point your knees forwards and your fingers backwards, to give a wonderful stretch to the front of your body, and to your arms and legs. Keep your hips high and remember to breathe slowly and smoothly.

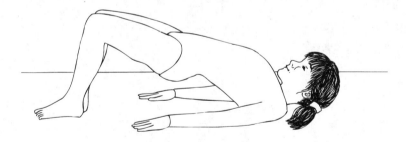

Figure 29 Bridge

ᐢᐢᐢ

CAMEL (DROMEDARY)

How to do it

1. Kneel down with your legs fairly close together and your toes pointing backwards. Breathe slowly and smoothly.
2. Support the small of your back (at the waist) with your hands; *carefully* tilt your head backwards.
3. *Slowly and carefully* place your right hand on your right heel and your left hand on your left heel. Keep your hips high. Imagine the curve of your body to be the hump of a camel (Figure 30).
4. Stay in this posture for as long as you comfortably can, remembering to breathe smoothly.
5. *Very slowly and carefully* return to your starting position.
6. Sit or lie down and rest.

What it does

The *Camel* strengthens your back and keeps your spine flexible. It keeps the organs in your abdomen (tummy) healthy (such as your bladder). It helps to keep your waistline trim. It keeps your hip and thigh muscles firm.

Special notes

This exercise has always been known as the *Camel*, but a better name would be 'dromedary'.

Dromedaries are light, fast-moving camels with one hump. They are bred for riding and carrying burdens. They are found in African and Arabian deserts.

Caution If you suffer from neck pain or have a serious back problem, it is best *not* to try this exercise.

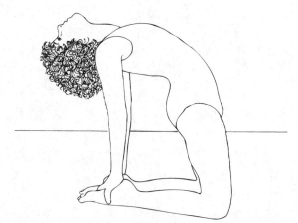

Figure 30 Camel (Dromedary)

CANDLE

How to do it

1. Lie on your back. Bend your knees and rest the soles of your feet flat on the mat. Keep your arms stretched out, close to your sides. Breathe slowly and smoothly.
2. Bring first one knee, then the other, to your chest.
3. Straighten one leg at a time until your feet point upwards.
4. Kick backwards *with both feet* at the same time, until your hips are off the mat. Support your hips with your hands, keeping your thumbs in front.
5. Gradually move your hands, one by one, towards your upper back, until your body is as straight as you can hold it comfortably (Figure 31).
6. Imagine that your body is a tall, straight candle, and your shoulders the candlestick; or you may wish to think of yourself as a candle on a birthday cake. Stay in this posture, breathing smoothly, until you are ready to come out of it.
7. Tilt your feet slightly backwards and put your arms down on the mat. Keep your head firm on the mat. Slowly lower your body, from top to bottom, onto the mat. Bend your legs, one at a time, and lower them to the mat. Rest.

What it does

The *Candle* is an excellent exercise to do for all-over health. It improves the look of your skin and hair, and is wonderful for your circulation.

Special notes

Try to include this exercise, or the *Half-Candle* (Figure 50), in your daily exercise programme, especially if you stand a great deal during the day. Because it is an inverted, or upside-down, posture, the *Candle* is a good balance to long periods of being on your feet.

Cautions If you have neck pain or an ear or eye problem, it is best *not* to try this exercise.

Girls should *not* practise this when they are having a period.

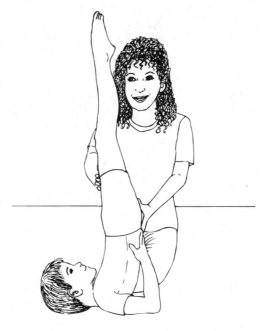

Figure 31 Candle

🚶🚶🚶🚶🚶🚶🚶🚶🚶🚶🚶🚶🚶🚶🚶🚶🚶🚶🚶🚶🚶🚶🚶🚶🚶🚶🚶🚶🚶🚶🚶🚶🚶🚶🚶

CHAIR

How to do it
1. Stand tall, with your feet comfortably apart. Breathe slowly and smoothly.
2. Stretch your arms out in front of you. Bend your knees, as if to sit. Keep your upper body straight (Figure 32).
3. Now you are a chair: your lower legs are the legs of the chair; your thighs form the seat; your body is the back, and your arms are the arm-rests. Stay in this posture for a few seconds. Continue breathing smoothly.
4. Stand up again.
5. Sit or lie down and rest.

What it does
The *Chair* is good for improving your balance and co-ordination, for strengthening your legs, and for keeping your ankle, knee and hip joints from becoming stiff.

Special note
To help you to keep your balance while doing this exercise, fix your gaze on some object in front of you, such as an ornament, a picture or a door handle. Breathing in and out slowly and smoothly also helps.

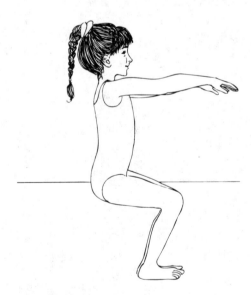

Figure 32 Chair

CHEST EXPANDER

How to do it

1. Stand tall, with your feet separated, but not too far apart. Keep your arms relaxed at your sides. Breathe slowly and smoothly.
2. As you inhale, raise your arms sideways to shoulder level; turn your palms downwards.
3. Exhale and lower your arms; swing them behind you and interlock the fingers of one hand with those of the other. Keep standing tall.
4. With your fingers still interlocked behind you, raise your arms to a comfortable height; keep them straight. Gently bend your head and body backwards (Figure 33).
5. Remain in this posture for as long as you comfortably can. *Do not* hold your breath.
6. Straighten your body. Lower your arms, unlock your fingers and relax.

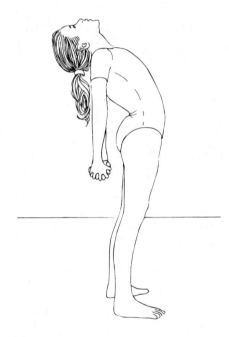

Figure 33 Chest Expander

𝍖𝍖𝍖𝍖𝍖𝍖𝍖𝍖𝍖𝍖𝍖𝍖𝍖𝍖𝍖𝍖𝍖𝍖𝍖𝍖𝍖𝍖𝍖𝍖𝍖𝍖𝍖𝍖𝍖𝍖𝍖𝍖𝍖𝍖

What it does

The *Chest Expander* is superb for ridding your upper back and shoulders of built-up tension. It encourages good posture. It promotes deep breathing by expanding your chest. Deep breathing is good for the health of your whole body.

This exercise also strengthens the large muscles that enable you to make powerful arm movements when swimming and rowing. These are the same muscles that you use in vigorous exhalation (breathing out) when singing.

Special notes

You can also practise the *Chest Expander* when sitting on a stool or bench. Do it any place where you can swing your arms freely behind you.

Practise this exercise in between classes at school; after sitting at a desk or computer for a long time, or after doing any activity that requires you to bend forwards for any length of time.

Bring some imagery into the exercise for added benefits: as you breathe in, imagine filling your mind and body with good, positive things such as courage, love and joy. As you breathe out, imagine sending away bad, negative things such as anger, disappointment and hatred.

COBRA

How to do it
1. Lie on your front or abdomen (tummy). Turn your head to one side. Rest your arms alongside your body. Breathe slowly and smoothly.
2. Turn your head to the front. Rest your forehead on the mat. Place your palms on the mat under your shoulders; keep your arms close to your body.
3. Inhaling, bend backwards *very slowly and carefully*: first, touch the mat with your nose, then your chin; then continue the backward bend in one smooth movement until your body becomes a graceful arch. Keep your hips on the mat (Figure 34).
4. Stay in this posture for as long as you comfortably can. *Do not* hold your breath.
5. *Slowly* return to your starting position in reverse: first, lower your abdomen to the mat; next your chest, then your chin, nose and forehead.
6. Turn your head to the side, relax your arms beside you and rest.

What it does
This is a splendid exercise for helping to keep your spine flexible and healthy. It also exercises the joints of your shoulders, elbows and wrists, keeping them strong and easy to move.

When you are in the completed *Cobra* posture, and breathing smoothly, the organs inside your abdomen receive a gentle massage, which helps to rid your body of wastes.

Special notes
The *cobra* is a poisonous snake found in India and Africa. When it becomes excited, its neck widens and flattens, and looks like a hood.

The *Cobra* posture is also part of the *Sun Greeting* exercises (Figure 20).

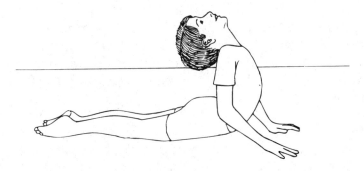

Figure 34 Cobra

𐅃𐅃 𐅃𐅃

COMPLETE RELAXATION

How to do it

1. Lie on your back. Separate your legs. Keep your arms away from your sides; turn your palms upwards. Close your eyes. Breathe slowly and smoothly throughout the exercise (Figure 35).

2. Push your heels away from your body; bring your toes towards you. Keep your feet like this for a few seconds. (From now on, this step will be referred to as 'hold'). Let go of the tightness you feel in your ankles and legs. Let the full weight of your legs and feet sink into the mat.

3. Tighten your buttocks (bottom). Hold the tightness for a few seconds. Release it; let go of the tightness. Relax your hips.

4. *Exhale* and press the back of your waist (also called the 'small of the back') against the mat. Feel your abdominal (tummy) muscles tighten. Hold. Release the tightness as you inhale. Relax your abdomen.

5. *Inhale* and squeeze your shoulderblades together. Hold for a few seconds while breathing smoothly. Release the squeeze as you exhale.

6. Shrug your shoulders, as if to touch your ears with them. Hold. Release the shrug.

7. *Carefully* tilt your head backwards. Feel the front of your neck stretch *gently*. Hold. Release the stretch.

8. *Carefully* tilt your head forwards, tucking in your chin. Hold. Untuck your chin. Make your head comfortable.

9. Raise your eyebrows, as if you are surprised. Feel your forehead wrinkle. Hold. Unwrinkle your forehead.

10. Squeeze your eyes shut tightly. Hold. Release the squeeze.

11. *Exhale* and open your eyes very widely. Open your mouth; stick your tongue out. Tighten all the muscles of your face. Look as fierce as you can, like a hungry lion (Figure 55). Inhale and relax the muscles of your face. Pull your tongue in. Close your mouth. Close your eyes. Continue breathing smoothly.

12. Stiffen your arms and raise them off the mat. Make tight fists. Hold. Rest your arms on the mat again. Relax them. Relax your hands.

13. Turn your thoughts to your breathing. Inhale. Fill your body with air. Feel your abdomen rise. Exhale. Let the air out. Feel your abdomen fall and relax. Continue breathing slowly and smoothly. Each time you inhale, imagine filling your body with good things, like love and peace and happiness. Each time you exhale, let your body sink more heavily into the mat. Let go of tightness in your muscles. Be completely relaxed from top to toe.

14. When you are ready to get up, turn on to your side and get up *very slowly*. Leisurely stretch your fingers, your arms and your legs. Yawn if you feel the need to do so. Wriggle your toes. *Never* jump up suddenly after relaxing completely.

What it does

Complete Relaxation is one of the best ways of ridding yourself of built-up tension, that feeling of being 'uptight'. It calms you down when you feel anxious or in a panic. It gives you energy when you are tired.

Special notes

Use any imagery with which you feel comfortable in step 13 of the instructions. You may wish, for example, to visualize yourself lying on a warm, sandy beach in summer, with a gentle breeze touching your face and hair, as you think happy thoughts.

Ask a parent, teacher or friend to read the instructions for *Complete Relaxation* slowly into a tape recorder, or do so yourself. Listen to the recording whenever you need to relax fully.

Practise this exercise when you come home from school, to give you energy for after-school activities, and to help you to stay calm. Practise it before you go to bed at night to help you to sleep soundly. Practise it in bed or in a comfortable chair when you are unwell. Change the instructions to suit the situation.

Always choose a quiet place in which to practise *Complete Relaxation*; find somewhere where you will not be interrupted for at least ten minutes.

Parents may find it helps to calm down a young child by doing *Complete Relaxation* together, using appropriate visualization as required.

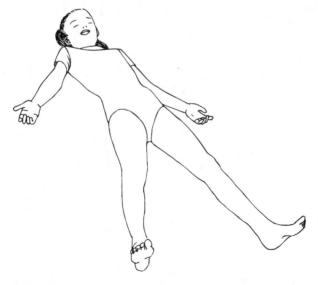

Figure 35 Complete Relaxation

COW HEAD

How to do it

1. Sit on your heels, in the *Japanese Sitting Position* (Figure 51). Breathe slowly and smoothly.
2. Reach over your right shoulder with your right hand. Keep your arm close to your ear and point your elbow straight upwards, like the horn of a cow.
3. With your left hand, reach behind your back *from below*. Interlock the fingers with those of your right hand. Remain sitting tall (Figure 36).
4. Stay in this posture for as long as you wish.
5. Return to your starting position.
6. Repeat steps 2 to 4, this time with your left hand over your left shoulder, and your right hand reaching behind your back from below.
7. Return to your starting position. Rest.

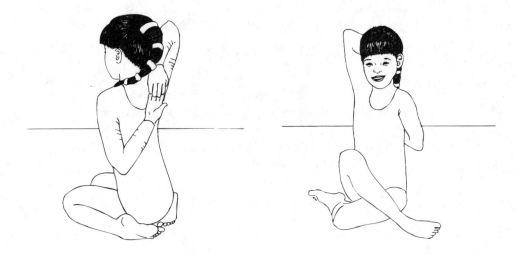

Figure 36 Cow Head   **Figure 37** Cow Head – variation

Variation

In this version of the *Cow Head*, your legs are bent and crossed, with one knee above the other, and your feet are beside your hips or thighs (Figure 37). The rest of the exercise is the same as described in steps 2 to 6 above. When the right knee is uppermost, the right elbow should point upwards, and when the left knee is uppermost, the left elbow should point upwards.

What it does

Practising the *Cow Head* posture regularly keeps the joints of your shoulders and arms flexible. It helps you to develop good posture. It relaxes tight chest muscles, and so helps you to breathe more deeply and release stale air from your lungs. It leaves you feeling refreshed and calm.

Special notes

Practise this exercise several times every day. It is especially useful after you have been bending over a desk, or sitting in front of a computer screen for a long time.

In the variation of the *Cow Head*, the crossing of the legs helps to keep your knee and hip joints flexible as well.

CROW

How to do it

1. Begin by squatting (see Figure 65), but place your feet wide apart, and your arms between your legs. Breathe slowly and smoothly.
2. Gently, but firmly, push against your arms with your legs, and push against your legs with your arms.
3. Rest your palms on the mat. Spread your fingers wide apart, and pretend that they are a crow's feet.
4. Slowly, carefully and with full attention, shift your weight onto your hands, until both feet lift off the mat at the same time. To help you to keep your balance, move your body as a single unit, and do not hang your head down (Figure 38). Keep breathing smoothly.
5. Now you are a crow on a perch. Stay in this posture for as long as you can.
6. Return to your starting position. Rest.

What it does

The *Crow* is an excellent exercise for developing balance, co-ordination and concentration. It strengthens your arms, wrists and fingers.

Special notes

If you wear glasses, take them off before trying the *Crow*. When first attempting this exercise, place a folded blanket, a cushion or a pillow in front of you to protect your face, in case you tip over.

It is important to concentrate on what you are doing when practising this and other balancing exercises. Keeping your attention on slow, smooth breathing helps you to do this.

The *Crow* is easier to do than it seems at first. Keep trying.

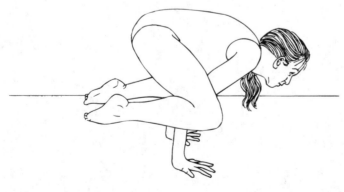

Figure 38 Crow

ﾊﾊ ﾊﾊ

CURLING LEAF

How to do it
1. Sit in the *Japanese Sitting Position* (Figure 51). Breathe slowly and smoothly.
2. Bend forwards and rest your forehead on the mat; or turn your head to the side.
   Rest your arms and hands beside you; turn your palms upwards (Figure 39).
3. Stay still, like a leaf curled up on the ground, for as long as you wish.
4. Go back to your starting position.

What it does
The *Curling Leaf* gives a wonderful stretch to your spine and to the muscles of
your back. It is also a very good way in which to relax. Do it following exercises
such as the *Bow* (Figure 28), the *Camel* (Figure 30), the *Cobra* (Figure 34), the
Fish (Figure 46), the *Swan* (Figure 68) and the *Wheel* (Figure 75).

As you breathe smoothly while doing this exercise, the organs in your body
receive a gentle massage. This is good for your blood circulation and for
removing wastes from your body.

Special notes
If at first your forehead does not touch the mat, put a pillow or cushion in
front of you, on which to rest your head.

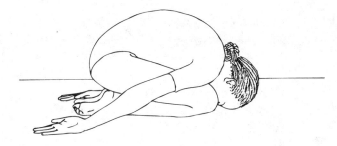

Figure 39 Curling Leaf

CURL-UP

How to do it

1. Lie in your back. Stretch your legs out and separate them a little. Breathe slowly and smoothly.
2. Bend your knees, slide your feet towards your bottom and rest your feet flat on the mat. Keep them in this spot for the rest of the exercise.
3. Rest your palms on your thighs.
4. Exhale as you *slowly and carefully* raise your head and shoulders. Keep your eyes fixed on your hands. Slide your hands along your legs, as if reaching for your knees. When you feel your abdominal (tummy) muscles tighten as much as you can comfortably bear it, stop there (Figure 40).
5. Breathe smoothly as you stay in this posture for as long as you can, *without strain*.
6. Ease yourself back onto the mat, from bottom to top, into your starting position. Rest.

What it does

The *Curl-Up* is superb for developing firm abdominal muscles. Firm, strong abdominal muscles are important for the health of your back and spine.

Special notes

It is not necessary to touch your knees in this exercise; just reach for them.

If you wish to try a diagonal version of this exercise, reach towards the outside of your left knee with both hands; then repeat this to the other side, to balance the stretch.

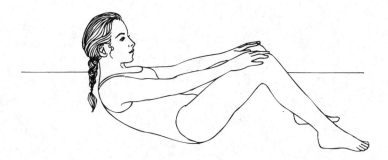

Figure 40 Curl-Up

DANCER'S POSE

How to do it

1. Stand tall, with your feet a little apart, and your body weight distributed equally between them. Breathe slowly and smoothly.
2. Shift your weight onto your *right* foot. Pay attention to your breathing; it will help you to keep your balance.
3. Bend your left leg, hold the foot with your left hand and bring it close to your bottom.
4. Raise your *right* arm straight upwards (Figure 41).
5. Stay in this posture for as long as you are comfortable in it.
6. Go back to your starting position. Rest.
7. Repeat the exercise, this time standing on your *left* foot, and raising your *left* arm. Rest afterwards.

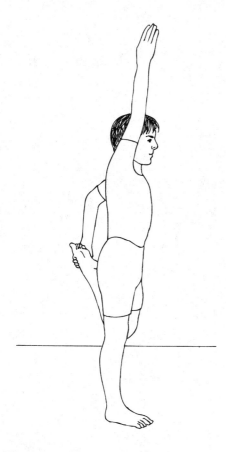

Figure 41 Dancer's Pose

Variation
In this version of the *Dancer's Pose*, you *slowly and carefully* bend forwards. Still holding the foot of the bent leg, push it away from your bottom (Figure 42).

What it does
The *Dancer's Pose* and its variation are splendid exercises for helping you to develop good balance, co-ordination and concentration. They exercise the large muscles at the front of our upper legs (called the *quadriceps*). These muscles are used for straightening your knees.

Special notes
If you fix your gaze on an object, such as a door handle or a picture on a wall, while doing the *Dancer's Pose* and other balancing postures, it will help you to keep steady. Concentrating on your slow, smooth breathing is also helpful.

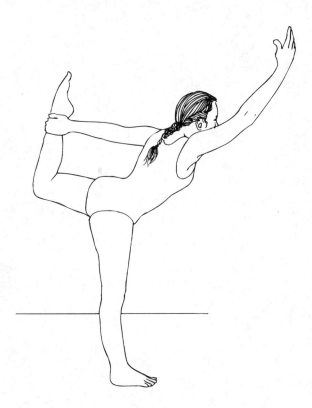

Figure 42 Dancer's Pose – variation

DOG STRETCH

How to do it

1. Start in an 'all fours' position on your hands and knees. Your arms should slope forwards. Breathe slowly and smoothly.
2. Tuck your toes in, so that they point forwards. Rock backwards slightly. Raise your knees and straighten your legs (Figure 43). Straighten your arms. Look downwards. Aim your heels towards the mat, but *be careful not to strain* the muscles at the back of your legs (the hamstrings).
3. Imagine you are a dog stretching its legs and body, to wake itself up after a nap. Stay in this posture for as long as you are comfortable in it.
4. Gently rock forwards before returning to your starting position.
5. Sit on your heels in the *Japanese Sitting Position* (Figure 51).
6. Rest in the *Curling Leaf* posture (Figure 39).

What it does

The *Dog Stretch* is a very good exercise to do to prevent your hamstring muscles from becoming tight and short. (The hamstring muscles are at the back of your thighs. They bend your knees and extend your thighs. When the hamstrings shorten, backache can result.)

This exercise brings a fresh supply of blood to your face and scalp, and therefore helps to keep your skin and hair healthy.

Special note

The *Dog Stretch* is part of the *Sun Greeting* exercises (Figure 21).

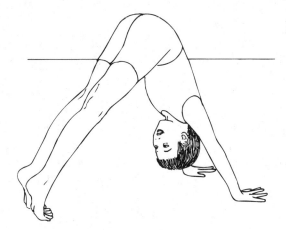

Figure 43 Dog Stretch

EAGLE

How to do it

1. Stand tall, with your arms at your sides. Breathe slowly and smoothly.
2. Slowly lift your *right* foot; pay full attention in order to keep your balance.
3. Cross your right leg over your left; hook the toes around your lower left leg. Keep breathing smoothly, and stand as tall as you can.
4. Bend your *right* arm and hold it in front of you.
5. Bend your left arm and place it inside the bent right arm; rotate your wrists until the palms are together (Figure 44).
6. Imagine yourself to be an eagle, perched high on a mountain top, guarding its nest. Stay in this posture for as long as you comfortably can.
7. Slowly unfold your arms, then your leg, and go back to your starting position. Rest for a few seconds.
8. Repeat the exercise, this time standing on your right foot, and placing your bent right arm inside your bent left arm.

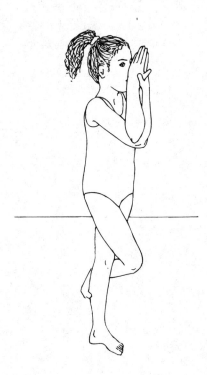

Figure 44 Eagle

Variation
In this version of the *Eagle*, you bend forwards (Figure 45), as if to swoop down to catch a fish for dinner.

What it does
The *Eagle* gives you a chance to exercise all the joints of your arms and legs. This prevents stiffness, and keeps the joints flexible.

Since it is a balancing exercise, the *Eagle* also helps to improve your co-ordination, concentration and alertness.

Special notes
If you fix your gaze on a still object, such as a plant or a picture on a wall, while doing the *Eagle* or any other balancing posture, it will help you to keep steady. Concentrating on your slow, smooth breathing is also helpful.

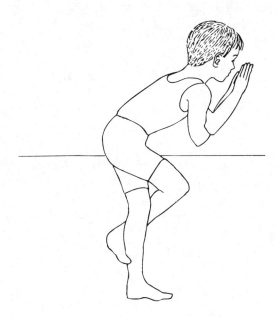

Figure 45 Eagle – variation

FISH

How to do it

1. Lie on your back. Stretch your legs out in front, and keep your arms beside you. Turn your palms down. Breathe slowly and smoothly.
2. Bend your arms. Push down on your elbows as you raise your chest and arch your back.
3. *Carefully* slide your head towards your shoulders. Rest the top of your head on the mat. Feel your neck stretch gently. You should take most of your weight on your bottom and elbows; *not* on your head and neck (Figure 46).
4. Close your eyes for a few moments and imagine that you are a fish floating. Breathe slowly, smoothly and deeply. Stay in this posture for as long as you are comfortable in it.
5. *Slowly and carefully* ease yourself back into your starting position. Rest.

What it does

The *Fish* is a splendid exercise to practise regularly if you suffer from asthma, or if you are anxious. It enables you to breathe deeply, and it helps you to relax.

Special note

The *Knee Press* (Figure 53) is a good posture in which to rest and relax your back after doing the *Fish*.

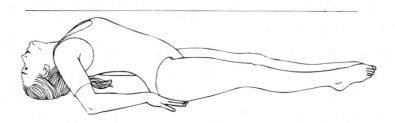

Figure 46 Fish

FLOWER

How to do it

1. Sit tall, in a folded-legs posture (Figures 56 to 58) or in the *Japanese Sitting Position* (Figure 51). Breathe slowly and smoothly.
2. Hold your hands in front of you; make fists, like tightly-closed flower buds.
3. Very *slowly* and with fingers kept stiff, open your hands, like sleeping buds unwillingly unfolding to the bright rays of the morning sun (Figure 47). Keep breathing smoothly.
4. When your hands are wide open, like a flower in full bloom, give your fingers a final stretch until they arch backwards. Stretch your arms sideways, if you wish.
5. Lower and relax your arms and hands.

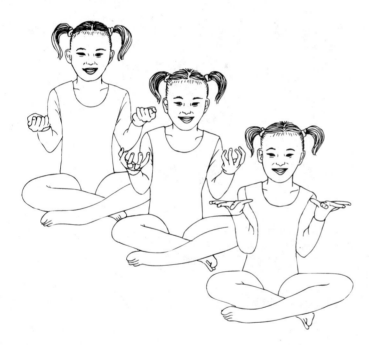

Figure 47 Flower

What it does
The *Flower* is excellent for improving the blood circulation to your hands and fingernails. It helps to rid your hands of tension, and it keeps your fingers supple. It is a splendid exercise if you use your hands a great deal – to write, draw, paint, sew, play a musical instrument, and so on.

Special notes
You may practise the *Flower* sitting on a bench, stool or log, or in a standing position also.

After practising the *Flower*, shake your fingers vigorously, as if ridding them of drops of water. This will leave your hands feeling warm and relaxed.

GRASSHOPPER

How to do it

1. Lie on your abdomen (tummy), facing downwards, with your chin touching the mat. Keep your legs fairly close together. Keep your arms straight, under your body. Make fists and keep your thumbs down. (You can, instead, keep your arms straight alongside your body.) Breathe slowly and smoothly.
2. *Exhale* and slowly raise one still-straight leg as high as you comfortably can. Keep your chin, arms and body pressed to the mat (Figure 48).
3. Hold this raised leg posture for as long as you comfortably can, imagining yourself to be a grasshopper getting ready to jump. Breathe slowly and smoothly as you do so.
4. Slowly lower your leg to the mat. Rest.
5. Repeat steps 2 to 4 of the exercise, raising the other leg this time.

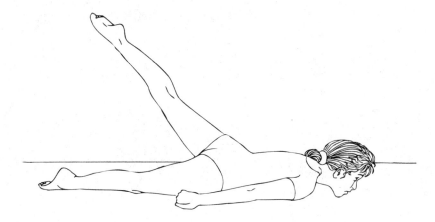

Figure 48 Grasshopper

Variation

In this version of the *Grasshopper*, you raise both legs while *exhaling* (Figure 49). You breathe as smoothly as you can while staying in the posture for as long as you comfortably can (Figure 49). Afterwards, you slowly lower your legs to the mat and rest.

What it does

The *Grasshopper* is very good for strengthening your back and legs. It also gives a gentle massage to your abdomen and the organs inside it, to help them to stay healthy.

Special notes

The *Grasshopper* is also called the *Locust*. Locusts are a type of grasshopper, mostly found in Africa. They sometimes gather together in countless numbers, and destroy all vegetation in their path.

Try resting in the *Curling Leaf* posture (Figure 39) after practising the *Grasshopper*. It will relax your back.

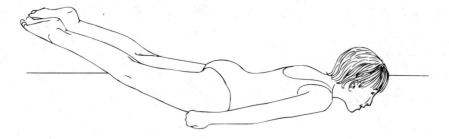

Figure 49 Grasshopper – variation

HALF-CANDLE

How to do it
1. Lie on your back. Bend your knees and rest the soles of your feet flat on the mat. Keep your arms close to your sides; turn your palms down. Breathe slowly and smoothly.
2. Bring one knee towards your chest; do the same with the other knee.
3. Straighten one leg at a time until your feet point upwards.
4. Kick backwards with both feet at once, until your hips are off the mat. Support your hips with your hands, thumbs in front (Figure 50).
5. Think of your legs as half of a tall candle, and your upper body as a candlestick. Stay in this posture for as long as you are comfortable in it. Continue breathing smoothly.
6. Put your hands back on the mat, one at a time.
7. Keep your head pressed to the mat and your chin up, and *slowly and carefully* lower your body from top to bottom onto the mat. Bend your knees and lower your legs to the mat, one at a time. Rest.

What it does
Like the *Candle* (Figure 31), the *Half-Candle* is an excellent exercise to do for all-over health. It is especially good for helping to keep your skin clear and your hair shiny.

Special note
Whereas your body is tall and straight in the *Candle* (Figure 31), it is tilted in the *Half-Candle*, to give the idea that the candle has burned down to the halfway mark.

Cautions If you have a neck pain or an eye problem, it is best *not* to do this exercise.

Girls should *not* practise this posture when they are having a period.

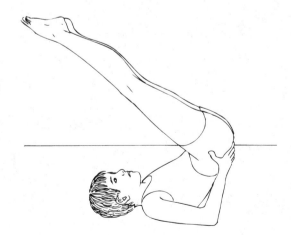

Figure 50 Half-Candle

JAPANESE SITTING POSITION

How to do it
1. Kneel with your legs together and your toes pointing backwards. Hold yourself tall. Breathe slowly and smoothly.
2. Lower yourself until you are sitting on your heels; use your hands to help, if necessary.
3. Rest your hands, palms down, on your thighs (Figure 51).
4. Sit in this posture for as long as you are comfortable in it.
5. Come out of the posture and rest.

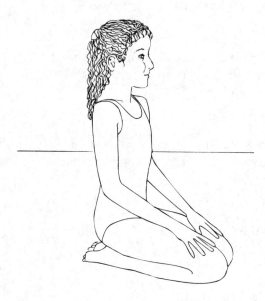

Figure 51 Japanese Sitting Position

♟♟♟

Variation

In this version of the *Japanese Sitting Position*, you start by kneeling, then you spread out your feet and sit on the mat between them, rather than sitting on the heels (Figure 52).

What it does

The *Japanese Sitting Position* gives you a solid, stable base on which to sit. It encourages you to be still and to stay calm. It is a good posture in which to sit when you practise breathing exercises, for example.

The *Japanese Sitting Position* also encourages good posture, which helps you to stay healthy and to feel confident.

Special note

See how many everyday things you can do in the *Japanese Sitting Position*, rather than sitting on a chair to do them.

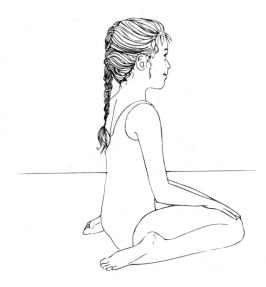

Figure 52 Japanese Sitting Position – variation

KNEE PRESS

How to do it

1. Lie on your back, with your legs stretched out in front. Rest your arms beside you. Breathe slowly and smoothly.
2. Bring first one bent knee, then the other, towards your chest or abdomen (tummy). Hold your knees or lower legs to keep them in place (Figure 53).
3. Stay in this posture for as long as you are comfortable in it. Keep breathing smoothly.
4. Stretch out one leg at a time. Relax your arms at your sides.

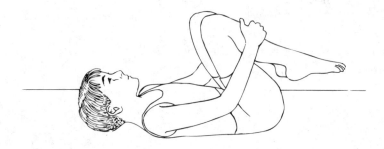

Figure 53 Knee Press

Variation
In this version of the *Knee Press*, you bring your forehead towards your knees (Figure 54).

Stay in this posture for as long as you comfortably can. Return to your starting position. Rest.

What it does
The *Knee Press* and its variation are splendid for relaxing your back muscles, and for getting rid of wind.

Special note
The *Knee Press* (Figure 53) is a good way in which to rest after doing backward-bending exercises like the *Bridge* (Figure 29), the *Fish* (Figure 46) and the *Wheel* (Figure 75).

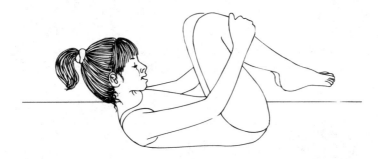

Figure 54 Knee Press – variation

LION

How to do it

1. Sit in the *Japanese Sitting Position* (Figure 51). Breathe slowly and smoothly.
2. Inhale. *Exhaling*, open your mouth widely and stick your tongue out. At the same time, open your eyes widely, as if staring. Tighten the muscles of your neck and face. Stiffen your arms and fingers. Now you are a fierce lion (Figure 55).
3. When you have no more air left to breathe out, pull in your tongue and close your mouth. Close your eyes. Relax the muscles of your neck, face, arms and hands. Breathe smoothly.

What it does

The *Lion* is a marvellous exercise for ridding your jaws of tension. Many people have tight jaws without realizing it. Tightness of the jaws can lead to headaches and to dental problems. Practising the *Lion* regularly can also help to improve the quality of your voice. In addition, it can help to prevent bad breath.

Special note

Practise the *Lion* several times during the day when you feel a sore throat coming. It can help to prevent it, or can make it less uncomfortable and help it to heal faster.

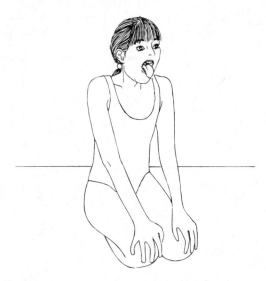

Figure 55 Lion

LOTUS

How to do it
1. Sit tall, with your legs stretched out in front. Breathe slowly and smoothly.
2. Cross your ankles. Bend your legs and pull the crossed ankles as close to your body as you can. Lower your knees towards the mat. Rest your hands on your knees or in your lap (Figure 56). This version of the *Lotus* is called the *Easy Pose*.
3. Sit like this as long as you wish. Close your eyes or keep them open. Think of yourself as a beautiful flower.
4. Stretch out your legs. Rest.

Variations
1. In this *Lotus* variation you start, as before, with your legs stretched out in front.
2. Bend your left leg and place the sole of the foot high up against your inner right thigh.
3. Bend your right leg and place the foot in the crease formed by the left calf and thigh. Rest your hands on your knees or in your lap (Figure 57). This version of the *Lotus* is called the *Perfect Posture*.
4. Sit like this for as long as you wish. Close your eyes or keep them open. Imagine that you are a pink water-lily in a clear pond.
5. After a while, you may change the position of your legs, so that the right leg is uppermost this time.
6. Stretch out your legs and rest.

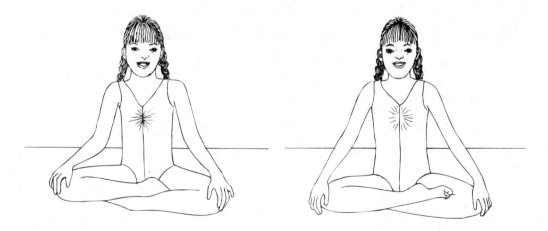

Figure 56 Lotus – Easy Pose   **Figure 57** Lotus – Perfect Posture

Full Lotus

1. Begin as before, by sitting with your legs stretched out in front.
2. Bend one leg and rest the foot high up on the opposite thigh.
3. Bend the other leg, and place the foot on the thigh of the opposite leg (Figure 58).
4. Sit like this for as long as you are comfortable in it. Close your eyes or keep them open. Think of yourself as a lotus flower.
5. After a while, change the position of your legs, if you wish.
6. Stretch out your legs and rest.

What it does

The *Lotus* poses give you a firm, stable base on which to sit for long periods. They encourage you to sit still and to stay calm. They are excellent postures in which to sit when practising breathing exercises. They are superb for developing good posture, which helps you to stay healthy and feel confident.

Special notes

The *Easy Pose* is known as 'tailor sitting'. It was a favourite of Indian tailors. It involves the large, ribbon-shaped muscles of the thigh, called the *sartorius* muscles (from the Latin word, *sartor*, which means 'tailor'). The sartorius is the longest muscle of the body, and helps to bend the knee.

The *Full Lotus* is a challenging version for students who are advanced and very flexible. *Do not force* your legs into this posture.

The *lotus* is an Indian water-lily with large pink petals.

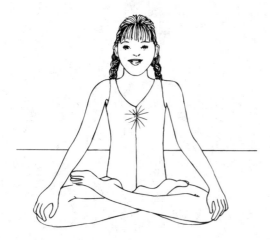

Figure 58 Full Lotus

LYING TWIST

How to do it

1. Lie on your back. Stretch your arms sideways, level with your shoulders. Breathe slowly and smoothly.
2. Bend your legs, one at a time, and rest the soles of your feet flat on the mat.
3. Bring your knees towards your chest.
4. Keeping your shoulders, arms and hands pressed to the mat, *slowly and smoothly* tilt your knees to one side as you *exhale* (Figure 59). You may turn your head to the side, opposite your knees, or you may keep it still.
5. Inhale and bring your knees back to the centre.
6. *Exhale* and tilt your knees to the other side.
7. Inhale and bring your knees back to the centre.
8. Continue this smooth side-to-side tilting of your knees, as many times as you wish.
9. Stretch out your legs, relax your arms and rest.

What it does

The *Lying Twist* is a very good warm-up exercise. It firms and strengthens the muscles of your back and abdomen (tummy), and it keeps your waist trim.

Special note

This exercise is a good warm-up to do before practising the *Triangle* (Figure 72) and the *Twist* and its variation (Figures 73 and 74).

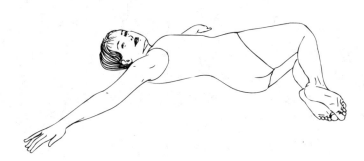

Figure 59 Lying Twist

MOUNTAIN

How to do it
1. Sit tall, in any comfortable cross-legged position, such as one of the
   Lotus postures (Figures 56 to 58). Breathe slowly and smoothly.
2. Inhale and stretch your arms overhead; keep them close to your ears. Point your
   fingers upwards and press your palms together. Keep your head level (Figure 60).
3. Close your eyes and pretend that your hands are the peak of a mountain,
   tall and strong, pointing towards the sky.
4. Remain in this posture for as long as you comfortably can.
   Keep breathing smoothly.
5. Lower your arms and relax your hands. Rest.

What it does
The *Mountain* helps to keep the muscles of your abdomen (tummy), back and
arms firm and healthy. It helps you to breathe more deeply, and it is also good
for your blood circulation.

Special notes
You can practise the *Mountain* standing, or in the *Japanese Sitting Position*
(Figure 51). You can also practise it sitting on a log, bench or stool.

Practise this exercise whenever you feel you need a good stretch,
such as after sitting at a desk or before a computer for a long time.

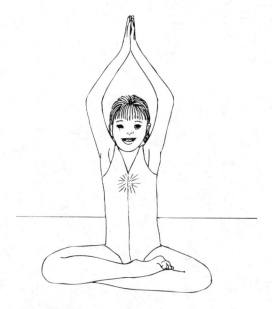

Figure 60 Mountain

PALMING

How to do it

1. Sit tall, at a desk or table, or any place where you can rest your elbows. Breathe slowly and smoothly.
2. First, briskly rub the palms of your hands together to warm them.
3. Place your palms *gently* over closed eyes, to shut out the light. Rest your fingers, kept close together, lightly on your forehead (Figure 61).
4. Stay in this posture for about a minute to start with. Keep breathing smoothly. Feel your eyes relaxing in the darkness.
5. Keep your eyes closed and repeat steps 2 to 4 for another minute, if you wish. If not, go on to step 6.
6. Spread your fingers apart and open your eyes to let the light in. Relax your arms and hands. Blink your eyes several times to end the exercise.

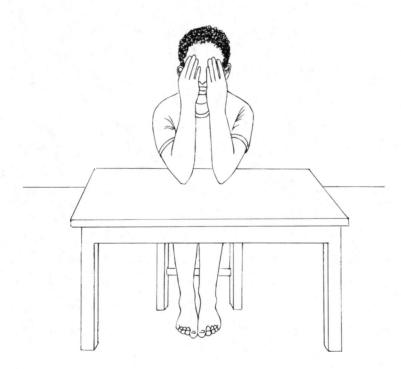

Figure 61 Palming

What it does
Palming, practised regularly, helps to prevent or to relieve eye strain. It is restful not only for your eyes, but also for your whole body. It improves concentration.

Special notes
Practise *Palming* from time to time during the day: after reading, writing and working with figures. Do it after sitting before a computer screen for a long time.

If you have nowhere to rest your elbows, you can still practise *Palming*, even while standing or lying down.

RABBIT

How to do it
1. Sit on your heels, with your toes pointing backwards. Breathe slowly and smoothly.
2. Lean forwards and rest your forehead on the mat, close to your knees.
3. *Carefully* raise your bottom off your heels, until the top of your head is resting *lightly* on the mat. *Do not press on your skull.* Hold on to your heels or ankles (Figure 62).
4. Stay in this posture for several seconds to start with; hold it longer as you are more comfortable with the exercise. Pretend that you are a rabbit taking a nap.
5. *Slowly* ease yourself back towards your heels. Keep your head low for a few seconds. *Slowly* sit up again and rest.

What it does
The *Rabbit* brings a fresh supply of blood to your head and face. It is therefore good for healthy skin and hair. It is also useful for helping you to relax.

Special notes
This exercise is sometimes called the *Hare*, which is a kind of rabbit. Have you ever read the story about the hare and the tortoise? If you have not, you might want to ask a parent, teacher or librarian to find it for you.

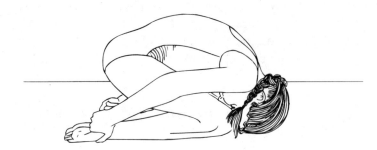

Figure 62 Rabbit

RAG DOLL

How to do it
1. Stand tall. Keep your arms at your sides. Breathe slowly and smoothly.
2. Tilt your head forwards, bringing your chin towards your chest.
3. Let your shoulders droop. Keep your arms and hands limp.
4. Slowly curl your body forwards. Allow the weight of your arms to pull your body downwards until it is hanging loosely. Let your arms dangle (Figure 63).
5. Now you are a floppy rag doll. Stay in this posture for as long as you wish. Breathe smoothly.
6. Slowly uncurl your body, from bottom to top, until you are standing upright again.
7. Sit or lie down and rest.

What it does
The *Rag Doll* is a splendid exercise for relaxing your whole body.

Special notes
The *Rag Doll* is a good cool-down exercise to do after practising the postures. It is also useful in helping you to relax at the end of the day, and to fall asleep easily at night.

When you are standing, loose and limp (step 5 of the instructions), imagine that all your tiredness is draining away from your body. Each time you exhale, pretend that you are sending away, with your breath, whatever may be troubling you. Each time you inhale, pretend that you are filling your body with health, courage and happiness. Use any imagery with which you feel comfortable.

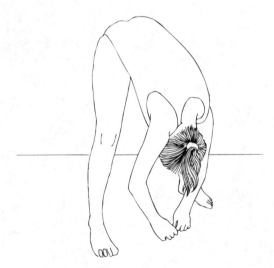

Figure 63 Rag Doll

SLIDE

How to do it

1. Sit tall, with your legs together and stretched out in front. Rest your hands on the mat behind you, fingers pointing away from your body. Breathe slowly and smoothly.
2. Press your palms down and raise your body. Keep your hips high. *Carefully* tilt your head back. Your weight should rest on your palms and feet (or heels). Your body, from neck to feet, should be straight, like a strong, smooth slide in a playground (Figure 64).
3. Stay in this posture for as long as you comfortably can. Keep breathing smoothly.
4. Lower your body to the mat and return to your starting position. Relax your arms and hands. Rest.

What it does

The *Slide* is a wonderful exercise for strengthening your body, legs and arms.

Special notes

Practise the *Slide* after back-stretching exercises such as the *Wheelbarrow* (Figure 76).

Please refer to the *Sun Greeting* exercises. Figure 18 (page 19) shows another 'slide', this time with the front of the body facing downwards.

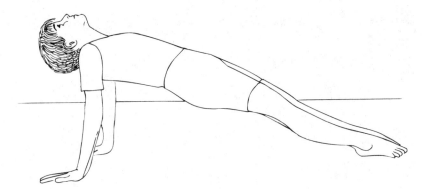

Figure 64 Slide

SQUAT

How to do it
1. Stand with your feet comfortably apart, and your arms at your sides. Breathe slowly and smoothly.
2. Inhale and raise your arms to shoulder level; rise onto your toes at the same time.
3. Exhale and slowly lower your arms; lower your body at the same time, as if to sit on your heels (Figure 65). Rest your feet flat on the mat, if you can.
4. Stay in this squatting posture for as long as you comfortably can. Breathe smoothly.
5. Return to your starting position. Sit or lie down and rest.

What it does
Squatting is superb for helping to keep your back healthy. It is excellent for keeping your ankle, knee and hip joints flexible. It is also useful for helping your body get rid of its wastes.

Special notes
See how many things you can do, every day, while squatting rather than standing or bending forwards. Some examples are: squat in a corner of the playground, park or beach to chat with a friend; squat to tidy a lower drawer of your chest of drawers; squat to polish your shoes.

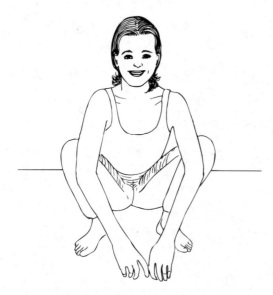

Figure 65 Squat

𑁋 𝕬𝕬𝕬𝕬𝕬𝕬𝕬𝕬𝕬𝕬𝕬𝕬𝕬𝕬𝕬𝕬𝕬𝕬𝕬𝕬𝕬𝕬𝕬𝕬𝕬

STAR

How to do it
1. Sit tall, with your legs stretched out in front. Breathe slowly and smoothly.
2. Bend one leg; place the sole of the foot beside the knee of the outstretched leg.
3. Bend your other (outstretched) leg; place the two soles together. Keep the feet in this spot throughout the exercise. Let your knees fall towards the mat.
4. Clasp your hands around your feet; hold them securely.
5. *Exhale* and slowly bend forwards; bring your face towards your feet. Relax your neck (Figure 66).
6. Stay in this posture for as long as you comfortably can. Close your eyes and breathe smoothly. Imagine that your head, knees and elbows are the five points of a star.
7. Ease yourself back into your starting position. Open your eyes. Rest.

What it does
The *Star* is a very good exercise for strengthening the inner muscle of your thighs and making them firm. It also helps to keep your hip, knee and ankle joints flexible. In addition, it keeps your spine and the muscles of your back healthy.

Special notes
Good exercises to do following the *Star* are the *Bridge* (Figure 29) and the *Slide* (Figure 64), both of which stretch the muscles on the opposite side of your body.

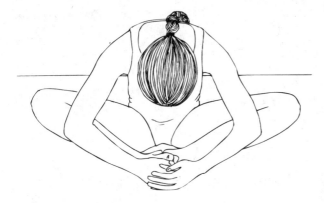

Figure 66 Star

STORK

How to do it
1. Stand tall, with your feet together. Breathe slowly and smoothly.
2. Shift the weight of your body to one foot. Bend the other leg and point the foot backwards. Raise your arms at your sides. Relax your wrists (Figure 67). If you prefer, keep your arms down and relaxed at your sides.
3. Now you are a stork standing on one leg. Your arms are your wings. Stay in this posture for as long as you are comfortable in it. Breathe smoothly.
4. Return to your starting position. Rest for a few seconds.
5. Repeat the exercise, this time bending your other leg. Sit or lie down and rest afterwards.

What it does
Like other balancing exercises, such as the *Eagle* (Figure 44), the *Stork* helps to improve your co-ordination and concentration, and to keep you alert.

Special notes
If you fix your attention on some object in front of you, such as a picture on a wall, or an ornament on a table, it will help you to keep your balance while you practise the *Stork*. Concentrating on your slow, smooth breathing will also help to keep you steady.

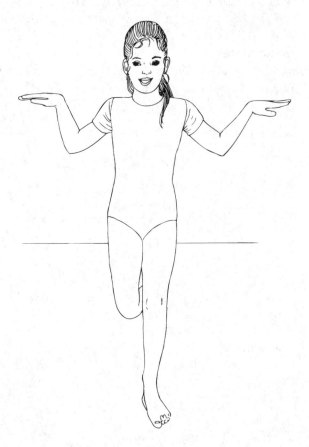

Figure 67 Stork

SWAN

How to do it

1. Lie on your abdomen (tummy). Turn your head to the side.
   Rest your arms alongside your body. Breathe slowly and smoothly.
2. Turn your head to the front. Rest your forehead on the mat. Place your
   palms under your shoulders; keep your arms close to your body.
3. *Inhaling*, bend backwards very *slowly and carefully*; first touch the mat
   with your nose then your chin; then continue the backward bend in one
   smooth movement, until your body becomes a beautiful arch. You are now
   in the *Cobra* posture (Figure 34).
4. Bend your legs and bring your feet towards your head. If you can, *carefully* tilt
   your head backwards a little more, and touch it with your feet (Figure 68).
5. Now you are a graceful swan, gliding on a lake that is calm and crystal-clear.
   Close your eyes and breathe smoothly. Stay in this posture only for as long
   as you are very comfortable in it.
6. Lower your legs to the mat. *Slowly* return to your starting position in reverse:
   first lower your abdomen to the mat; next to your chest, then your chin,
   nose and forehead.
7. Turn your head to the side, relax your arms beside you and rest.

What it does

This is a splendid exercise for helping to keep your spine flexible and healthy.
It also exercises the joints of your shoulders, elbows and wrists, keeping them
strong and flexible. The wonderful stretch the front of your body receives when
you practise the *Swan* helps to keep your abdomen firm and your waist trim.

Special note

The *Swan* is an advanced exercise. *Do not force* yourself into this position.
Try it only when your body has become very supple.

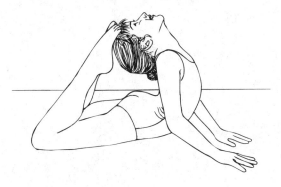

Figure 68 Swan

卂卂卂卂卂卂卂卂卂卂卂卂卂卂卂卂卂卂卂卂卂卂卂卂卂卂卂卂卂卂卂卂卂卂卂卂卂卂卂

TORTOISE

How to do it

1. Sit tall. Stretch your legs in front of you and spread them apart. Breathe slowly and smoothly.
2. Pull one heel towards you until the sole of the foot is flat on the mat. Do the same with the other heel.
3. Still holding yourself tall, bend forwards as you *exhale*, and reach out to touch your feet. Lower your head; relax your neck.
4. Bend your arms and pass them under your thighs. Turn your palms up (Figure 69). Breathe smoothly.
5. Once you are in this posture, straighten your legs out again as much as you can. *Do not strain.*
6. Stay in this posture for as long as you are comfortable in it. Close your eyes and pretend to be a tortoise: your body is the shell, and your arms and legs are the tortoise's feet.
7. To come out of the posture, bend your legs and bring your arms from under your thighs. Sit up again slowly before lying down to rest.

What it does

The *Tortoise* gives a wonderful stretch to your spine, legs and arms. It keeps these parts of your body fit and flexible.

Special notes

The *Tortoise* is sometimes called the *Turtle*. It is an advanced posture for people who have been exercising regularly for some time. *Do not strain* yourself in trying to do it.

Tortoises and turtles belong to a group of animals known as *chelonians*. Tortoises live on land, but most turtles live in water.

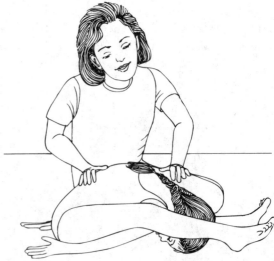

Figure 69 Tortoise

‽‽

TREE

How to do it
1. Stand tall, with your feet together and your arms at your sides. Breathe slowly and smoothly.
2. Lift one foot. Use your hands to help you place the sole of the foot high up against the inner thigh of the opposite leg.
3. Reach upwards with both arms. Press your palms together; point your fingers upwards (Figure 70).
4. Pretend to be a tall, strong fir tree. The foot on which you are standing is the main root that goes deep into the earth. Your legs and body are the trunk. Your arms are the branches, and your fingers the pointed top.
5. Stay in this posture for as long as you wish.
6. Return to your starting position. Rest for a few seconds.
7. Repeat the exercise, standing on the other foot this time.

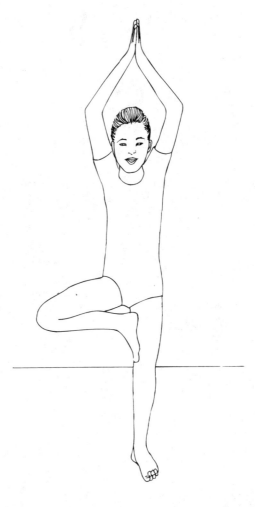

Figure 70 Tree

Variation

In this version of the *Tree*, the position of your feet is the same as before but your arms are held differently: stretch them out to the sides, like the branches of a spreading chestnut tree (Figure 71).

What it does

The *Tree*, like other balancing exercises such as the *Dancer's Pose* (Figure 41), is excellent for developing concentration, co-ordination and alertness.

Special notes

Keep your attention on some object in front of you, such as a door handle or a picture on a wall, to help you to remain steady. Concentrating on your slow, smooth breathing is also a good way to help you to keep your balance.

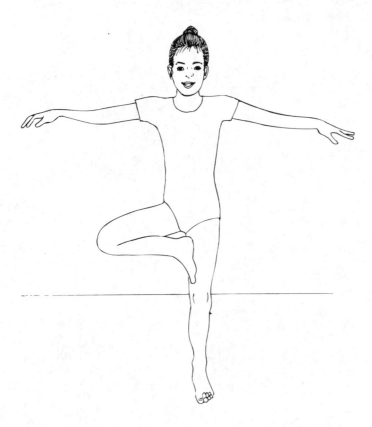

Figure 71 Tree – variation

TRIANGLE

How to do it
1. Stand tall, with your feet wide apart (about 24 inches, or 60 centimetres), and your arms at your sides. Breathe slowly and smoothly.
2. Inhale and raise your left arm; exhale and bend sideways to the right, sliding your right hand down the side of your right leg. Take care not to lean forward. Keep your left arm alongside and above your ear (Figure 72).
3. Stay in this posture for as long as you are comfortable in it. Keep breathing smoothly.
4. Return to your starting position. Rest.
5. Repeat the exercise (steps 2 and 3), but this time raise your right arm and bend to the left.

What it does
The *Triangle* is excellent for keeping the muscles at the sides of your body, and those of your abdomen (tummy) firm and healthy. It helps to keep your waist trim and makes it easier for you to breathe deeply. Deep breathing is very good for your health.

Special note
A *triangle* is a figure bounded by three straight lines. This exercise takes its name from the fact that the completed posture looks like a triangle: your feet form the base, and your arms and sides represent the other two sides of the triangle.

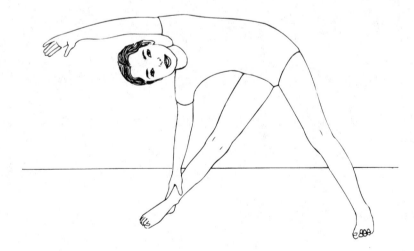

Figure 72 Triangle

TWIST

How to do it

1. Sit tall, with your legs stretched out in front of you. Breathe slowly and smoothly.
2. Bend your *left* knee and lift your left leg over your right leg. Rest your *left* foot on the mat near the *outside* of your right knee.
3. Exhale and *slowly and smoothly* twist your upper body to the *left*. Place both palms on the mat at your *left* side. Turn your head and look over your *left* shoulder (Figure 73).
4. Breathe smoothly. Close your eyes and imagine yourself to be a corkscrew (or perhaps a pretzel). Stay in this posture for as long as you are comfortable in it.
5. *Slowly and smoothly* untwist your body. Go back to your starting position.
6. Repeat the twist in the other direction: follow steps 2 to 4, but this time bend your *right* knee, and twist your body to the *right*.
7. *Slowly and smoothly* untwist. Return to your starting position. Rest.

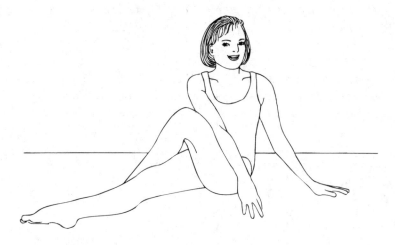

Figure 73 Twist

Variation

In this version of the *Twist*, you fold the straight leg inwards (Figure 74).
The rest of the exercise is the same as before.

What it does

This is the only yoga posture which requires maximum twisting of your spine,
first to one side then to the other. This is excellent for keeping your spine flexible,
and for looking after the health of the organs located in this part of your body,
such as your kidneys.

Special note

Here is a tip which will help you to remember to which side to twist your body
and turn your head: when your *left knee is up, twist to the left*. When your *right
knee is up, twist to the right*.

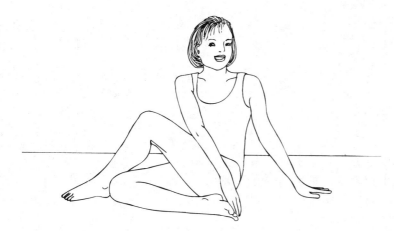

Figure 74 Twist – variation

WHEEL

How to do it

1. Lie on your back, with your legs stretched out and your arms at your sides. Turn your palms down. Breathe slowly and smoothly.
2. Bend your legs and rest the soles of your feet as near to your bottom as you comfortably can.
3. Raise your arms and pretend to make a half-circle with them, until they are behind your shoulders. Rest your palms on the mat, with your fingers pointing towards your shoulders.
4. Press on your hands and feet, and *slowly and smoothly* raise your body to form a graceful curve, like that of a wheel (Figure 75).
5. Keep breathing smoothly. Stay in this posture for as long as you are comfortable in it.
6. *Slowly and carefully* ease yourself out of the posture, in reverse, until you are again lying flat on the mat.
7. Stretch out and rest. Relax your arms at your sides.

What it does

The *Wheel* gives a wonderful stretch to your legs, arms and front of your body. It helps to keep your spine flexible and healthy. It widens your chest to help you to breathe more deeply.

Special note

Try the *Wheel* only if you are already very fit and flexible. *Do not strain.* This is a posture which provides a challenge for advanced students.

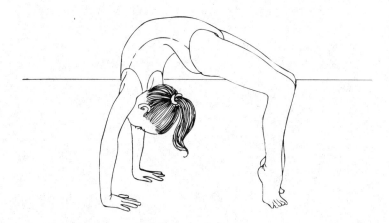

Figure 75 Wheel

WHEELBARROW

How to do it

1. Lie on your back, with your legs stretched out and close together. Rest your arms beside you. Turn your palms down. Breathe slowly and smoothly.
2. Bend your legs and bring your knees to your chest. Straighten your legs so that your feet point upwards.
3. *Exhale* and kick both feet backwards at the same time, until your hips are off the mat.
4. Lower your feet back over your head; try to touch the mat with them. Keep your legs together, if you can, and as straight as possible (Figure 76). *Do not let your hips go past your shoulders, as this could strain your neck.*
5. Breathe smoothly. Close your eyes and pretend that you are a wheelbarrow: your body is the barrow itself, and your feet are the handles. Stay in this posture for as long as you comfortably can.
6. Ease yourself back onto the mat, in reverse. Bend your legs and lower them to the mat. Rest.

What it does

The *Wheelbarrow* is superb for keeping your back healthy and your spine flexible. It is also useful for helping your body to get rid of its wastes.

Special note

This exercise is also known as the *Plough*. You may not have seen an old-fashioned plough, but it is still used in some countries. It is a farming tool, sometimes drawn by oxen or horses, which is used to cut the soil and turn it up before planting.

Caution Girls should *not* practise this posture when they are having a period.

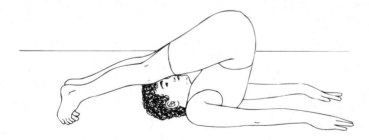

Figure 76 Wheelbarrow

†† ††

Chapter five

Breathing Exercises

THE ACT OF BREATHING, which is known as *respiration*, consists of two movements: *inhalation*, or breathing in, and *exhalation*, or breathing out. In quiet breathing, the *diaphragm* does most of the work. The diaphragm is a dome-shaped muscle, inside your body, which separates your chest from your abdomen (stomach). When you inhale, the diaphragm contracts, or grows smaller, and causes your chest to enlarge from top to bottom. At the same time, contraction of your chest muscles causes your chest to enlarge from back to front and from side to side. Your lungs then expand, or grow larger, to fill this increased space, and air is drawn into the air passages leading to your lungs.

When you exhale, air is forced out by relaxation of the muscles, and by the elastic recoil, or springing back, of the lungs, similar to the way in which a stretched rubber band springs back when the stretch is released. To help you to understand this action better, think of your chest as a hand holding a sponge (the lungs) in water: when your hand opens, the sponge expands, and when your hand closes, the sponge is squeezed.

Your breathing and your blood circulation work closely together. When you inhale, you take in oxygen from the outside. It passes through your nose, down your windpipe, and into your lungs. You need a constant supply of oxygen for your brain, muscles, and every other part of your body to do their work properly. You cannot live without oxygen.

The oxygen in the air you inhale is transferred to your blood. Your heart pumps the blood, which is rich in oxygen, to every part of your body by means of a network of blood vessels.

After the blood has circulated through your body, it returns to your heart as oxygen-poor blood. Your heart pumps it through your lungs where it picks up oxygen, to be circulated again throughout the body. In this way the entire circulation process repeats itself; it is a never-ending *circle* (think of the name, circulation).

When you exhale, you breathe out a waste product called *carbon dioxide*.

Your respiratory (breathing) system must be working well in order that your blood can pick up oxygen in your lungs. This is one reason why deep breathing and other exercises for improving respiration are so beneficial to your health. There is another health benefit to be gained from breathing slowly, smoothly and deeply, and that is the ability to stay calm when you are under pressure. This is because of the close relationship between your emotions, or feelings, and your breathing.

You can think of your state of mind, or how you feel, as a kite. Imagine that your breathing is the string that is attached to the kite, which controls it. When you are calm and happy, your breathing is slow and smooth, like the gentle, steady pull of the string. The kite will then glide and soar gracefully, like a carefree bird. When you are tense or troubled, however, your breathing is shallow and sometimes jerky, and you may even be short of breath. This is like the tugging of the kite string. It will cause the kite to pitch and toss, like a boat on rough seas, and get out of control.

Health benefits

Breathing and blood circulation work very closely together, so regular practice of the special exercises in this chapter will improve the oxygen supply to your body's organs and muscles, to give them the energy needed to do their work well.

Learning to exhale thoroughly helps you to rid your body of wastes, such as carbon dioxide. Controlling the length of your exhalation is also useful in helping conditions such as anxiety and asthma.

Because the way in which you breathe affects your emotions, or how you feel inside, learning to breathe slowly, smoothly and deeply, and doing so when you feel tense and worried, will be useful in helping you to keep calm and confident.

Rules to follow

1. When practising breathing exercises, always sit or stand tall, but *not stiff*. If you are lying down, try to relax as much as you can (*see* Figure 35, *Complete Relaxation*).
2. Keep your jaws, face, hands and body relaxed.
3. Unless you are instructed otherwise, breathe through your nostrils, with your mouth closed, but *not* tightly shut, so that the air may be warmed, moistened and filtered before reaching your lungs.
4. Inhale slowly, smoothly and as deeply as you can, *without strain*.
5. Exhale slowly, smoothly and as completely as you can, *without strain*.
6. *Do not* hold your breath at any time.

The following breathing exercises have been selected carefully because they are safe for children to do and they can be fun to practise. Parents and teachers working with younger children can make games out of the exercises, to hold their attention longer and to help their concentration to improve. Examples of such exercises are *Complete Breathing*, the *Humming Bee* and the *Runner's Breath*.

CALMING BREATH

How to do it
1. Sit tall. Keep your hands still. Close your eyes if you wish, or if it is safe to do so.
2. Inhale slowly and smoothly through your nostrils, and as deeply as you can without straining.
3. Exhale steadily through your nostrils. Fix your attention on your navel ('tummy button').
4. *Before inhaling again,* mentally count 'one thousand', 'two thousand'.
5. Repeat steps 2 to 4, again and again, until you feel calm.
6. Breathe slowly and smoothly without counting.

What it does
This breathing exercise is excellent for calming you down when you feel anxious, upset or about to panic.

Special notes
Help a friend or relative become calm again: tell him or her what to do, step by step, as in the instructions above.

You can do the *Calming Breath* lying or standing. You can do it almost any time or anywhere, such as before an exam, audition or interview, or before you see your dentist. No one will know what you are doing.

You can use imagery to help while doing this exercise. As you inhale, imagine filling your body and mind with good things, such as happiness, courage and hope. As you exhale, imagine sending away bad things, such as fear, sadness and disappointment.

COMPLETE BREATHING

How to do it

1. Sit tall, in any comfortable seated posture, such as the *Japanese Sitting Position* (Figure 51), or one of the *Lotus* poses (Figures 56 to 58). Keep your hands still. Close your eyes, if you wish. Breathe slowly and smoothly.
2. *Inhale* (breathe in) smoothly. Imagine filling the top of your lungs with air, then the middle, and then the bottom. As you do so, your chest will expand (widen) and your abdomen (tummy) will grow larger (Figure 77).
3. *Exhale* (breathe out) smoothly: imagine emptying your lungs, from top to bottom. As you breathe out, your abdomen will flatten and your chest will relax (Figure 78).
4. Repeat steps 2 and 3 several times: smooth, deep inhalation followed by smooth, complete exhalation.
5. Rest.

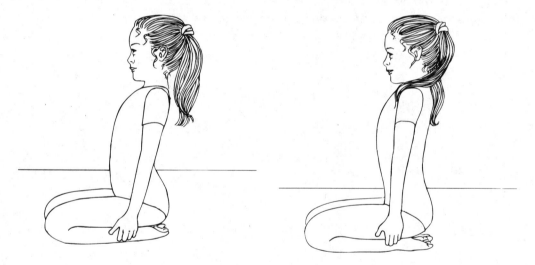

Figure 77 Complete Breath – inhaling   **Figure 78** Complete Breath – exhaling

What it does
Practising the *Complete Breath* regularly trains you to use your chest muscles, and other muscles involved in breathing, in the best possible way. It allows you to rid your body of more stale air than usual, and it enables a better supply of oxygen to reach your lungs and blood circulation. Practising the *Complete Breath* every day is one way of helping yourself to stay healthy.

Special notes
You may practise this breathing exercise standing up or lying down. If lying down, try placing a paper boat or airplane, or a small plastic duck on your abdomen, and note how it rises as you inhale and falls as you exhale.

If you rest your hands on your waist, with your palms down and your middle fingers touching each other, you will note that the fingers separate as you breathe in, and come together again as you breathe out.

To help you to remember this exercise, think of a balloon. As you put air into it, it becomes *fat*. As you let the air out, it becomes *flat*. In your mind, say the following: 'Air *in*, tummy *fat*. Air *out*, tummy *flat*'.

COOLING BREATH

How to do it

1. Sit tall, in any comfortable seated posture, such as the *Japanese Sitting Position* (Figure 51), or one of the *Lotus* poses (Figures 56 to 58). Keep your hands still. Close your eyes, if you wish. Breathe slowly and smoothly.
2. Stick your tongue out, and curl it lengthways to form a sort of tube (Figure 79). Inhale slowly and steadily through this 'tube'.
3. Pull your tongue in again; close your mouth and exhale through your nostrils.
4. Repeat steps 2 and 3 again and again, as many times as you wish.
5. Breathe in your usual way.

What it does

This is a useful breathing exercise to practise when your body is overheated, such as when you have a fever or when the weather is hot.

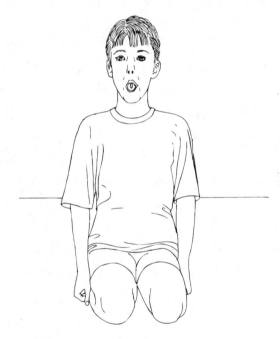

Figure 79 Cooling Breath

HUMMING BEE

How to do it
1. Sit tall. Unclench your teeth; relax your jaws. Keep your lips together, but *not tight*. Keep your hands still. Close your eyes. Breathe slowly and smoothly through your nostrils.
2. When next you *exhale*, say 'Hm-m-m-m', like a bee humming. Let the humming continue until you have no breath left.
3. Inhale slowly, smoothly and deeply again.
4. Exhale and make a humming sound, until your exhalation is complete.
5. Repeat steps 3 and 4, again and again, for a minute or two.
6. Breathe slowly and smoothly without humming.

What it does
The *Humming Bee* soothes the mind and body. Practise it after you have been in a very busy place and need a few quiet moments. Practise it when you feel troubled. It will help to relax and comfort you.

Special note
Give your full attention to the humming. This is what helps to pull your thoughts away from the hustle and bustle, and to make you feel calm.

RUNNER'S BREATH

How to do it
1. Sit tall, in the *Japanese Sitting Position* (Figure 51), or in any other comfortable seated posture. Keep your hands still. Close your eyes or keep them open. Breathe slowly and smoothly through your nostrils.
2. Next time you are ready to *exhale*, do so briskly, as if to sneeze. You will feel your abdomen (tummy) tighten and flatten.
3. Relax your abdomen. You will then be able to inhale naturally.
4. Repeat steps 2 and 3 a few times, to give you a good idea of what is happening: a brisk outward breath followed by a normal inward breath.
5. Repeat steps 2 and 3 again and again, at a faster pace: abdomen tightening on a brisk exhalation, and relaxing on inhalation.
6. Rest while breathing as usual.

What it does
The *Runner's Breath* trains you to use the muscles involved in breathing in the best possible way. It helps you to get rid of waste products from your body. It tones up your stomach muscles. Because it trains you to control your exhalation, this exercise is also useful for anyone who suffers from asthma.

Special notes
This breathing exercise is called the *Runner's Breath* because the quick pace of breathing reminds you of the way a runner breathes at the end of a race.

It is sometimes called the *Bellows Breath* because the quick, jerky way in which it is done sounds like a bellows in action. A *bellows* is an implement used for driving a blast of air into a fire. By expanding and collapsing, the bellows draws air through a valve, and forces it out to give a draught to the fire.

SIGHING BREATH

How to do it
1. Sit tall. Keep your hands still. Keep your eyes open or close them.
2. Inhale slowly, smoothly and deeply through your nostrils.
3. Exhale steadily through pouted lips, as if whistling or cooling a hot cup of tea or other drink. Close your mouth when you have no breath left.
4. Repeat steps 2 and 3, again and again, as many times as you wish.

What it does
The *Sighing Breath* is a good exercise to practise when you are tense, anxious, afraid or upset. It prevents these feelings from becoming worse, and it helps to make you feel calm.

Special note
You can practise this breathing exercise lying down or standing up. You can practise it almost anywhere: between classes, in a car or bus, or wherever you feel comfortable doing it.

SNIFFING BREATH

How to do it
1. Sit tall. Keep your hands still. Keep your eyes open or close them.
2. Instead of trying to take one long, deep inhalation through your nostrils, take three or four small, inward sniffs, as if breaking up the inhalation into small parts.
3. Exhale steadily through your nostrils.
4. Repeat steps 2 and 3, again and again, until you feel your chest relaxing, and you are able to take one slow, deep inward breath without straining.

What it does
The *Sniffing Breath* relaxes your chest muscles. It is the exercise of choice when you are so tense, and your chest is so tight, that you are unable to breathe in deeply. It also helps to relax your whole body.

Special notes
You can practise the *Sniffing Breath* lying or standing. You can practise it anywhere you feel comfortable doing it.

Babies and very young children sometimes do a sort of *Sniffing Breath* after they have been very upset, and before going to sleep. They take a series of short, quick inward breaths, followed by a long exhalation, after which they relax and breathe normally again.

WOODCHOPPER

How to do it

1. Stand tall, with your feet wide apart and your arms at your sides. Breathe slowly and smoothly.
2. Bring your arms in front and clasp your hands together, as if holding an imaginary axe.
3. *Inhale* and raise your arms upwards and backwards, with your hands still clasped. Pretend that you are raising your 'axe' as you prepare to chop a large piece of wood.
4. *Exhale* and swing your arms forwards, bringing your 'axe' downwards, between your legs, to 'chop the wood' (Figure 80).
5. Repeat steps 3 and 4 two or more times, until there is 'no more wood to chop'.
6. Return to your starting position. Breathe smoothly. Rest.

What it does

The *Woodchopper* is a powerful breathing exercise. It expands your chest to help you to breathe more deeply. It gets rid of more stale air from your lungs than when you are breathing in your usual way. It exercises your body to keep it strong and flexible.

Special notes

If you are upset or cross about something, practise the *Woodchopper* to help to get rid of angry feelings. As you bring your arms downwards while exhaling, imagine that you are getting rid of whatever is bothering you: send these thoughts away with your breath.

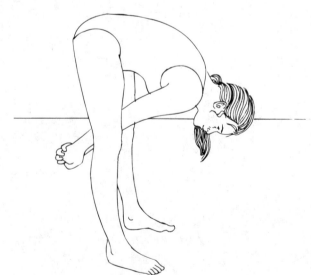

Figure 80 Woodchopper

Chapter six

Food for Fitness

Introduction

PARENTS, TEACHERS AND OTHER ADULTS responsible for the health and welfare of
children and young adults can do a great deal to foster, early in life, an awareness
of the importance of good nutrition. Children are not usually interested in what
is 'good' for them and what is involved in healthy eating. Teaching children about
foods that build life-long health, in an interesting and enjoyable way, can therefore
be a challenge! But it is one well worth taking up.

The information in this chapter is presented with the hope that it will help to
spark children's interest in the kind of foods that will help them to grow up
healthy and be mentally and physically fit.

The human body needs substances called *nutrients*, which are obtained from
the food we eat, to stay alive and healthy, and to do its work well. There are six
important classes of nutrients: water, proteins, carbohydrates, fats, vitamins and
minerals. They work together in teams.

Water

You need water to grow, and to stay alive and healthy, just as the plants and flowers
in a garden do. Water forms a major part of your blood, and it is by means of water
that nutrients are carried to every part of your body. Water is essential for your food
to be digested well, and for removing wastes from your body. It is also important for
keeping your temperature normal.

You can obtain water from all drinkable liquids, but fruit and vegetable juices,
herbal teas, milk and plain water are best. Most fruits have a high water content
and are therefore also a good source.

Proteins

Proteins are used to build new tissue and repair damaged cells. Your hair, skin, nails, eyes and muscles are made of protein.

Sources of animal protein include eggs, fish, meat, milk, milk products and seafood. Vegetable proteins can be obtained from bean sprouts, whole grains such as rice, legumes, which are dried beans, peas and lentils, as well as nuts, seeds and tofu, which is a soya bean product.

Carbohydrates

Carbohydrates are starches and sugars. They provide you with energy and help you to digest and use the food you eat. The chief source of your brain's energy is, in fact, the sugar that comes from carbohydrates.

The best sources of carbohydrates are carob powder, fresh fruits and vegetables, fresh fruit and vegetable juices, dried fruits, honey, pasta, whole grains and whole grain cereals.

Fats

Fats are important for forming healthy body cells, especially those needed for digestion and good memory. They are needed to provide energy and body heat, and also for sending the proper signals from your nerves to your muscles. They are necessary for certain nutrients to be properly absorbed, and they help to make food taste good.

Good sources of fat include butter, cheese, eggs, milk, nuts, and oils from vegetables, nuts and seeds, such as avocados, peanuts and sesame seeds.

Vitamins

Vitamins are substances necessary for life, and for your body to do its work well. You need vitamins for growth and energy, and you can obtain them in small quantities from wholesome food.

Here are the names of the important vitamins, what they are useful for, and where to obtain them.

Vitamin A

This vitamin is important for healthy eyes and good eyesight. It helps to prevent and fight infections. It is needed for growth, and for strong bones, healthy hair, teeth and gums, and for clear skin.

The best sources of vitamin A include fresh vegetables, especially the deep green and yellow ones such as broccoli, carrots, dandelion leaves, parsley, spinach, squash (or marrow), sweet potatoes and turnip tops. Vitamin A is also provided by fresh fruits, especially apricots, cantaloupe melons, cherries, mangoes, papaya and peaches. In addition, you can obtain this vitamin from butter, milk and milk products, egg yolk, fish liver oils, oily fish and liver.

The B vitamins

The B vitamins are a group, or 'complex', of more than twenty vitamins that are especially important for a healthy nervous system, and for clear skin, shiny hair and strong nails. They are also necessary to help to prevent and fight infections.

Good sources of the B vitamins include green leafy vegetables such as dandelion leaves, lettuce and spinach, as well as legumes and whole grains and cereals. Many breakfast cereals are enriched with the B vitamins. They are also found in fish and in meat such as liver.

All the B vitamins are essential and work together. The following three, however, are particularly important for children and young people.

Vitamin B_1, called *thiamine,* is needed for good appetite and for helping food to digest properly. It is useful in fighting car, air and seasickness. It keeps the nervous system and all muscles, including the heart, working well. It helps to keep you feeling cheerful.

You can obtain this vitamin from cantaloupe melons, green leafy vegetables such as spinach, and from legumes, oatmeal, peanuts, potatoes, sunflower seeds and whole grains.

Vitamin B_2, known as *riboflavin,* is important for growth and for healthy skin, hair and nails. It helps to relieve tired eyes, and to prevent a sore mouth, lips and tongue. It is needed for digesting food properly, and for obtaining energy from food.

Good sources of this vitamin include almonds, cantaloupe melons, cottage cheese, fish, green leafy vegetables such as lettuce and spinach, and also milk and sunflower seeds.

Vitamin B₃, also called *niacin*, is important for food to be digested and used properly, so as to provide energy. It is needed for clear, healthy skin and for preventing bad breath. It also helps to prevent dizziness and to heal canker sores.

Good sources of this vitamin include avocados, dates, eggs, figs, fish, green leafy vegetables, legumes, nuts, potatoes and wholewheat products.

Vitamin C

Vitamin C is important for helping to prevent and to fight infections (such as winter colds) and allergies, and to heal wounds. It is needed for a substance called *collagen*, which is a sort of glue that holds together the body's cells – forming tissues such as skin and bone. It is also needed for healthy blood circulation.

The following are among the best sources of vitamin C: fresh fruits such as apricots, berries of all kinds, cantaloupe and honeydew melons, cherries, grapefruit, guavas, kiwi fruit, kumquats, lemons, limes, oranges, strawberries, and rose hips which are the seed pods of roses (underneath the buds). Vitamin C is also obtained from fresh vegetables such as cabbage, dandelion leaves, green and red peppers, mustard and cress, potatoes and turnip tops.

Vitamin D

Vitamin D is necessary for strong bones and healthy teeth, and works together with vitamins A and C to help prevent colds.

The best sources of this vitamin include butter, eggs, herring, fish oils, milk enriched with vitamin D, salmon, sardines and tuna. (The body can also make its own vitamin D with the help of sunlight – simply from being outside in the sunshine.)

Vitamin E

Vitamin E is necessary for providing energy and preventing fatigue. It also helps to protect your lungs against pollution.

The best food sources of this vitamin include almonds and other nuts, broccoli, Brussels sprouts, eggs, fresh fruits, green leafy vegetables, legumes, seeds, soya beans, vegetable oils and whole grains and cereals.

Vitamin F

This vitamin, also known as *unsaturated fatty acids*, is needed for growth, and for healthy skin and hair. It is, in fact, needed for health in general.

The chief food sources of vitamin F are nuts, seeds and vegetables, and oils obtained from sources such as almonds, avocados, peanuts, soya beans, sunflower seeds and walnuts.

Vitamin K

Vitamin K is also known as 'the blood vitamin'. It helps to prevent excessive bleeding by helping blood to clot properly after cuts, scrapes or surgery.

The best food sources of this vitamin include alfalfa sprouts, egg yolk, fish liver oils, green leafy vegetables, milk and yogurt.

Vitamin P

Vitamin P helps to prevent bruising by strengthening the small blood vessels in your body, known as *capillaries*. It also helps to prevent your gums from bleeding, and strengthens your body to prevent and fight infections. It helps vitamin C to do its work well.

The best sources of vitamin P include the white skin and pulp of citrus fruits such as lemons, oranges and grapefruit, and also apricots, cherries, rose hips and strawberries.

Minerals

Minerals are the essential parts of all cells forming the greater portion of the hard tissues of your body, such as bones, nails and teeth.

Here are the names of some important minerals, what they are useful for, and where to obtain them.

Calcium

Calcium is necessary for strong bones and healthy teeth. It is important for your nervous system to work well, and for your heart to beat regularly. It helps you to sleep soundly at night, and to have strength and energy for your work and studies.

The best food sources of calcium include milk and milk products, blackstrap
. molasses, carob powder, citrus fruits, dried beans, dried figs, green vegetables,
peanuts, salmon, sardines, sesame seeds, soya beans, sunflower seeds and walnuts.

Iron

Iron is important for preventing *anaemia*, which is often called 'iron-poor blood'.
It increases your energy by preventing fatigue. It brings healthy colour to your
cheeks. It helps you to grow, and it helps to prevent and fight disease.

Good sources of iron include apricots, asparagus, blackstrap molasses, Brussels
sprouts, cauliflower, dried fruits, egg yolk, kiwi fruit, green leafy vegetables, nuts,
oatmeal, seeds, Sharon fruit (persimmon), strawberries, watermelon, whole grains
and whole-grain products, as well as lean red meat, liver, shellfish and sardines.

Magnesium

Magnesium works with calcium. It is necessary for energy, and for nerves and
muscles to do their work well. It is useful in preventing stomach aches caused by
indigestion. It helps to keep your teeth healthy. It is also needed for your heart and
blood vessels to work properly. In addition, magnesium helps to prevent you from
feeling depressed, and keeps you cheerful.

The best food sources of magnesium include alfalfa sprouts, almonds and other
nuts eaten fresh from the shell, apples, beetroot tops, blackstrap molasses, brown
rice, celery, dried fruits, grapefruit, green leafy vegetables such as spinach, lemons,
oranges, peas, potatoes, sesame seeds, soya beans, sweetcorn, whole grains and
whole-grain products.

Potassium

Potassium works with *sodium* (salt) in your body to keep your heart beating
regularly, and your body fluids in normal balance. It helps to improve your ability
to learn by sending more oxygen to the brain. It also helps your body to get rid of
its wastes. In addition, potassium helps to relieve allergies, colic and diarrhoea.

The best food sources of this mineral include bananas, citrus fruits, green leafy
vegetables such as lettuce and spinach, and also legumes, mint leaves, nuts,
potatoes, watercress, watermelons and whole grains and cereals.

Zinc

Zinc is like a a traffic police officer, seeing over and directing the workings of the inside of your body. It helps to increase mental alertness and your ability to learn. It improves your appetite and your sense of taste. It helps you to grow and to stay healthy. It prevents white spots from appearing on your fingernails, and it speeds up the healing of scrapes, cuts and other wounds.

Foods rich in zinc include cheese, eggs, broad beans (also called lima beans), green beans, mushrooms, non-fat dried milk, nuts, onions, pumpkin seeds, soya beans, sunflower seeds and whole-grain products. Zinc is also to be found in liver and shellfish.

Top ten nutrients

Like pop records, nutrients have their own 'top ten'. Not counting water, they are: proteins, carbohydrates, fats, vitamin A, vitamin B_1 (thiamine), vitamin B_2 (riboflavin), vitamin B_3

(niacin), vitamin C, calcium and iron.

As a general rule, if you are obtaining enough of these nutrients from wholesome food, you are likely to be getting enough of the other important nutrients also.

Wise choices

With so many foods from which to choose, it is sometimes difficult to make healthy choices. The following suggestions are therefore offered to help you to select foods and drinks that build up health rather than break it down.

- Drink water, fresh fruit and vegetable juices, milk and milk shakes and herbal teas instead of colas and other soft fizzy drinks.
- Eat carob products, low in sugar, instead of chocolate and sweets.
- For snacks, eat fresh fruits, low-salt crackers and crispbreads made from whole grains, cheese, hard-boiled eggs, raw vegetables, yogurt and dried fruits (brush your teeth afterwards). Nuts, pumpkin and sunflower seeds and popcorn also make good snacks, but *do not* give them to children under five years of age, as they may choke on them.

Word List (Glossary)

THE WORD GLOSSARY comes from the old Greek word *glossa*, which first meant 'tongue' and later 'word'. Now it means 'a collection of explanations'.

Here are explanations of some of the words used in this book.

Abdomen	Stomach (tummy) or belly. Part of the body, between the chest and the hips.
Abdominal	Refers to the abdomen.
Alert	Watchful, attentive, or observant.
Allergy	Over-sensitiveness to some foreign food or protein, or to some substance that does not normally cause a reaction (such as dust or cat hair).
Angle	Space between two lines or surfaces, where they meet.
Anti-clockwise	Moving in a curve from right to left. *Anti* means 'opposite' or 'against'. 'Clockwise' means going from left to right, following the direction of a clock's hands.
Asana	Yoga exercise. Posture or pose.
Audition	A trial hearing, test or performance. From the Latin word *audire*, which means 'to hear'.
Balance	Steadiness. Keeping steady.
Beneficial	Helpful. Valuable or good for.
Benefit	Help, good or of value. To benefit is to be useful or to do good for someone or something.
Bibliography	List of books. List of references.
Blackstrap molasses	A product of sugar refining. Also called treacle or molasses. A thick, dark, sticky liquid rich in vitamins and minerals.
Bladder	A sac, such as the *urinary bladder*, which stores urine in the body.
Blood circulation	*See* Circulation.

Calf muscle	Muscle at the back of the leg, below the knee.
Canker sore	Sore of the mouth and lips.
Carbon dioxide	A gas given off by the body, through the lungs.
Carob powder	A powder (or flour) made from the ground seed pods of the locust tree. Looks and tastes a bit like cocoa or chocolate.
Carefree	Free from care or worry.
Caution	Carefulness. Concern for safety. Warning.
Cells	Tiny units which make up all body parts.
Challenge	Something that tests a person's qualities or skills.
Chief	Main, principal or leading. Most important.
Choice	Preference, selection or pick.
Circulation	A circular course, such as that of the blood throughout the body. Blood is circulated in the body by means of the heart and blood vessels.
Citrus fruits	Group of fruits including grapefruit, lemons, limes, oranges and tangerines.
Colic	Pain, either steady or occurring on and off, usually in the abdomen (tummy).
Concentrate	Give full attention.
Concentration	The act of giving full attention to something.
Confident	Sure of oneself.
Content	The content of something is that which it contains.
Contract	Draw together or reduce in size. To contract a muscle is to draw it together so it shortens.
Control	Power to direct, rule, manage or regulate.
Co-ordination	Working together to produce a certain movement.
Dental	Refers to the teeth.
Depressed	Low in spirits. Very sad.
Diagonal	Running from corner to corner, in a slanting direction.
Diarrhoea	Frequent loose stools (bowel movements).
Digestion	The breaking down of food for use by the body.
Disappointment	Let-down. Feeling of failure or defeat.
Disease	Unhealthy condition of body or mind, or both. Sickness.
Distribute	Divide or share.
Dizziness	Sensation of whirling. Feeling about to fall. Giddiness.
Draught	Current of air.
Dromedary	Camel with one hump, used for carrying burdens, or for riding. Found in Arabian and African deserts.
Emotions	Strong feelings, such as fear, love, anger or happiness.
Essential	Necessary. Needed.
Excessive	Too much. Needless.

Exhalation	Act of breathing out. Opposite of inhalation.
Expand	Spread out. Widen. Increase in size.
Eye strain	Tiredness of the eye or eyes, due to over-use.
Fatigue	Tiredness. Weariness.
Filter	Strain, cleanse or purify.
Flexible	Able to bend without breaking. Easy to bend.
Forehead	Front part of the head, above the eyes, and below the hairline.
Gaze	A fixed look. To look long and steadily at something or someone.
Green leafy vegetables	The green leaves of certain vegetables, which can be eaten. Includes beetroot tops, dandelion leaves, lettuce, mustard and cress, spinach and turnip tops as well as broccoli etc.
Greeting	Expression or gesture used when meeting someone. A welcoming.
Guarding	Protecting or defending.
Hamstring muscles	Muscles on the back of the thighs, which bend the legs. Also called the *hamstrings*.
Hygiene	Practice of health rules.
Image	Picture. Mental picture.
Imagery	Images or pictures occurring in someone's mind.
Imaginary	Existing in the imagination. Made-up or make-believe.
Imagination	Creative thought. Power to form mental pictures.
Implement	Tool or instrument.
Indigestion	Improper breaking down of food in the body. It sometimes produces a stomach-ache.
Infection	Disease. Spread of disease or 'germs'.
Inhalation	Act of breathing in. Opposite of exhalation.
Instructions	Directions or explanations.
Interlock	Connect, lock or clasp two or more things together.
Interview	Question-and-answer meeting. A spoken examination of someone looking for employment.
Jerky	Having sudden movements. Not smooth.
Joint	The point where two or more bones meet.
Kidneys	Two organs in the back of the abdomen, which excrete, or get rid of, urine from the body.
Knowledge	Learning. Understanding.

Legumes	Dried beans, peas, lentils and peanuts.
Leisurely	Slow-moving. Relaxed. Not hurried.
Lengthways	In the direction of the length, that is, from end to end of the long side of something.
Level	Flat, even or smooth. In a smooth line.
Librarian	Person in charge of a library, or a member of the staff in a library.
Limber	Flexible or supple.
Locust	A type of grasshopper. Locusts are usually found in Africa and Asia. They sometimes gather in large numbers and destroy plants.
Lotus	The lotus is an Indian water-lily with large pink petals. The lotus poses are seated postures in yoga in which the legs are folded.
Lungs	Two cone-shaped spongy organs concerned with breathing. They are located in the chest.
Maintain	Continue. Go on with. Carry on with.
Major	Chief. Greater.
Massage	Rub-down. A firm rubbing of the muscles and joints of the body, with the hands.
Maximum	The greatest possible amount, number or degree.
Meditate	Think quietly. To fix your attention on only one thing or activity, shutting out everything else from your thoughts.
Mental	Refers to the mind.
Milk products	Foods made from milk, such as cheese, cottage cheese and yogurt.
Natural	Refers to something produced by nature, or existing in nature. Normal. Regular.
Navel	Small dent at the middle of the abdomen or stomach (tummy). 'Tummy button'.
Negative	Gloomy or dark. Opposite of positive.
Nervous system	The brain, spinal cord (running along the inside of the spine), and nerves branching off the spine.
Normal	Usual, general, habitual, ordinary or regular.
Nostrils	Openings in the nose, for breathing in and out.
Observe	Watch. Take notice of. Keep your eyes on.
Opposite	On the other or farther side. In the other direction.
Organs	Body parts, which perform special functions, for example, the heart.
Otherwise	Differently. In a different way.

Ox	A member of the cow family. (The plural of this word is *oxen*).
Oxygen	A colourless, odourless (without smell) gas. The air you breathe in contains oxygen, which is necessary for health and for staying alive.
Panic	A great fear of something, the cause of which is not always known. Terror or fright.
Parallel	At an equal distance from something at all points, and going in the same direction.
Pasta	Food products made with a 'paste' of flour and water (and sometimes also egg). These include lasagne, macaroni and spaghetti.
Peak	Pointed top, such as that of a mountain.
Perch	Something on which a bird rests, such as a bar in a cage, or a tree branch. A resting place.
Permission	Being allowed. Consent.
Physical	Refers to the body.
Pitch	Toss about. Rise and fall.
Pollution	State of being impure, unhealthy or unclean.
Popular	Liked or admired by people in general.
Positive	Bright. Confident. Opposite of negative.
Posture	How you hold and carry yourself. Also refers to yoga exercises.
Powerful	Strong.
Preparation	What you do to get ready for something.
Pressure	Stress. Strain. Difficulty.
Pretend	Make believe. Imagine.
Prevent	Stop from happening.
Privacy	Secret or hidden from others. Not disturbed by others. Quiet.
Proceed	Move forward. Carry on. Continue.
Product	Something produced, made or grown.
Progress	Forward movement. Movement nearer a goal. To progress towards something is to show improvement.
Promote	Help forwards. Encourage. Work towards. Help.
Prop	A support placed under or against something to hold it up.
Protect	Defend. Guard. Watch over. Look after.
Provide	Give. Offer. Supply. Yield.
Realize	Understand. Know.
Recoil	Spring back. Draw back. Shrink back.
Regular	Usual. Normal. Well-balanced. Even.

🕴🕴

Reinforce	Strengthen or support.
Relax	Be less tense. Loosen up. Take it easy.
Relaxation	State of being without unnecessary tension. Calm state. Rest from work.
Relieve	Free from something, such as pain or anxiety. Make something less.
Represent	Stand for. Serve as. Show a likeness of. Act the part of.
Respiration	The act of breathing in and out.
Result	End. Outcome. Product. Effect.
Reverse	Move backwards. Go in the opposite direction.
Rigid	Stiff. Not easy to bend. Tense.
Rose hips	Fruits of the rose. The seed pods of wild roses. The nodule (rounded lump) underneath the buds of roses (called 'hips').
Rotation	Movement in a circle. Turning. Twisting.
Scalp	The skin on the top and back of the head, to which hair is attached.
Second	A small measurement of time. There are sixty seconds in one minute.
Secure	Safe. Firm. Fixed. Tight. Firmly fastened.
Select	Choose or pick out.
Separate	Keep apart. Opposite of keep together.
Serpent	Snake.
Session	Period of time spent in some activity, such as doing exercises.
Shallow	Not deep.
Shift	Change or alter. Move from one place, position or condition to another.
Sigh	A deep outward breath that can be heard, to express relief, sadness or contentment.
Skid	Slip or slide. 'Non-skid' describes something that does not slip or slide, but stays in place.
Skull	Bony framework of the head.
Slope	Slant or lean. Not level.
Sneeze	Sudden and forceful outward breath, through the nose or mouth, usually with a loud noise.
Soar	Rise high into the air. Float high in the air.
Soles	Bottom of the feet. Also bottom of shoes.
Soothe	Calm, smooth, ease, comfort or relieve.
Source	Origin. Where something comes from or where it can be obtained.
Spare	Extra, additional or left-over.
Spine	Backbone.

Spreading	Stretching outwards, or opening out fully.
Stable	Secure, sound, solid, steady, fixed, firm or safe.
Strict	Exact or careful.
Suggestion	Idea, hint or advice.
Supple	Easy to bend. Flexible. Limber.
Support	Prevent from falling. Hold up. Strengthen.
Surface	Outside. Outer face. Covering.
Surgery	Operation. Treatment or work done by a surgeon.
Survival	Keeping alive.
Swoop	Come down, or descend, swiftly and suddenly.
Target	Any object at which something is aimed.
Temperature	Degree of heat. Hotness or coldness.
Tend	Likely to. Lean towards.
Tense	Highly-strung. Uneasy. Strained. 'Up-tight'.
Tension	Stress. Strain. Tightness. Pressure.
Thigh	Upper leg, between the hip and knee.
Tilt	Lean, slant or slope.
Tissue	A mass of cells or fibres, which make up parts of the body.
Tofu	A custard-like product made from soya beans. Soya curd or cheese.
Tone	Refers to the normal, healthy state of any part of the body. To tone up your muscles is to make them firm.
Toss	Move up and down, or back and forth jerkily.
Train	Teach or coach. To help someone reach a certain standard through instruction and practice.
Triangle	A figure with three sides and three angles ('tri' means 'three').
Trim	Fit, neat, lean or slim. In good condition.
Unclench	Loosen, open or relax. To clench your teeth is to press them closely together. Unclenching them is the opposite.
Unit	A single thing. Whole.
Unwilling	Not wanting. Opposed.
Upright	Erect. Straight up.
Usual	Normal in habit or practice. Ordinary. Regular.
Valve	A fold of membrane in a passage or tube in the body. It allows fluid to pass in one direction only.
Vegetation	Plant life in general.
Version	Creation. Presentation. Special or different form of something.
Vigorous	Energetic, strong, powerful or lively.

Visualization	The act of seeing something in your mind. Imagining. Forming pictures in your mind.
Warm-up	An exercise, or a period of exercise, done before a game or race, or before practising yoga postures.
Wastes	Products to get rid of. Material that is no longer useful.
Welcome	Greet. Receive warmly or eagerly.
Whole-grain products	Refers to products made from whole grains such as wheat, in which the bran (outer covering) and the germ (at the centre of the grain) have not been removed.
Wholesome	Healthy. Health-giving. Nourishing. Strengthening.
Yogi	Someone who practises yoga as a way of life.

Book List (Bibliography)

THE FOLLOWING WORKS were consulted, and found useful, during the research for this book.

A'nanda Ma'rga. *Teaching Asanas*, Los Altos Hills, California: Amrit Publications, 1973

Anderson, Bob. *Stretching*, Bolinas, California: Shelter Publications, 1980

Ballentine, Rudolph M., Jr. M.D. (Ed.). *Joints and Glands Exercises As Taught by Sri Rama of the Himalayas*, Homesdale, Pennsylvania: Himalayan International Institute of Yoga Science and Philosophy, 1973

Carr, Rachel. *Yoga for All Ages*, New York: Simon and Schuster, 1972

Davis, Adelle. *Let's Eat Right to Keep Fit*, New York: The New American Library, 1970

Lidell, Lucy, with Narayani and Giris Rabinovitch. *The Sivananda Companion to Yoga*, New York: Simon and Schuster, 1983

Mindell, Earl. *The Vitamin Bible for Your Children*, London: Arlington Books, 1981

Papastavrou, Vassili. *Wildlife at Risk. Turtles and Tortoises*, Hove, England: Wayland (Publishers), 1991

Plourde, Renée Guimond, RN, BScN. 'Le stress de l'Écolier', Ottawa, Canada: *The Canadian Nurse*, pp. 40-43

Purna, Dr Svami. *Balanced Yoga*, Shaftesbury, Dorset: Element Books, 1992

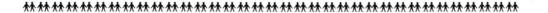

Sobol, Tom, and Sobol, Harriet. *Your Child in School. Kindergarten Through Second Grade,* New York: Arbor House, 1987
—*Your Child in School. The Intermediate Years: Grades Three Through Five,* New York: Arbor House, 1987

Stewart, Mary, and Phillips, Kathy. *Yoga for Children,* New York and London: Simon and Schuster, 1992

Swire, Susan. *Gentle Exercise,* London: J. M. Dent & Sons, 1986

Weller, Stella. *The Yoga Back Book,* London: Thorsons, 1993

Index